The Pool Activity Level (PAL) Instrument for Occupational Profiling

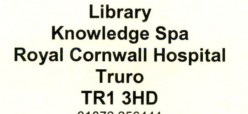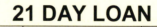

Bradford Dementia Group Good Practice Guides

Under the editorship of Murna Downs, Chair in Dementia Studies at the University of Bradford, this series constitutes a set of accessible, jargon-free, evidence-based good practice guides for all those involved in the care of people with dementia and their families. The series draws together a range of evidence including the experience of people with dementia and their families, practice wisdom, and research and scholarship to promote quality of life and quality of care.

Bradford Dementia Group offer undergraduate and postgraduate degrees in dementia studies and short courses in person-centred care and Dementia Care Mapping, alongside study days in contemporary topics. Information about these can be found on www.bradford.ac.uk/acad/health/dementia.

other books in the series

Involving Families in Care Homes
A Relationship-Centred Approach to Dementia Care
Bob Woods, John Keady and Diane Seddon
Bradford Dementia Group Good Practice Guides
ISBN 978 1 84310 229 8

Person-Centred Dementia Care
Making Services Better
Dawn Brooker
Bradford Dementia Group Good Practice Guides
ISBN 978 1 84310 337 0

Ethical Issues in Dementia Care
Making Difficult Decisions
Julian C. Hughes and Clive Baldwin
Bradford Dementia Group Good Practice Guides
ISBN 978 1 84310 357 8

Design for Nature in Dementia Care
Garuth Chalfont
Bradford Dementia Group Good Practice Guides
ISBN 978 1 84310 571 8

of related interest

Evaluation in Dementia Care
Edited by Anthea Innes and Louise McCabe
ISBN 978 1 84310 429 2

Dementia Care Training Manual for Staff Working in Nursing and Residential Settings
Danny Walsh
ISBN 978 1 84310 318 9

The Pool Activity Level (PAL) Instrument for Occupational Profiling

A Practical Resource for Carers of People with Cognitive Impairment

Third Edition

Jackie Pool

Jessica Kingsley Publishers
London and Philadelphia

First edition published in 1999 by Jessica Kingsley Publishers
Second edition published in 2002 by Jessica Kingsley Publishers

This edition published in 2008
by Jessica Kingsley Publishers
116 Pentonville Road
London N1 9JB, UK
and
400 Market Street, Suite 400
Philadelphia, PA 19106, USA

www.jkp.com

Library of Congress Cataloging in Publication Data

Pool, Jackie, 1957-
  The pool activity level (PAL) instrument for occupational profiling : a practical resource for carers of people with cognitive impairment / Jackie Pool. -- 3rd ed.
    p. cm.
  ISBN-13: 978-1-84310-594-7 (pbk. : alk. paper) 1. Dementia--Treatment. 2. Occupational therapy. 3. Dementia--Patients--Care. I. Title.
  RC521.P659 2008
  616.8'3--dc22
                        2007019934

British Library Cataloguing in Publication Data
A CIP catalogue record for this book is available from the British Library

ISBN 978 1 84310 594 7

Printed and bound in Great Britain by
Printwise (Haverhill) Ltd, Suffolk

Contents

Part 2 Using the Pool Activity Level (PAL) Instrument in Leisure Activities

Sarah Mould and Jackie Pool

About the Author and Contributors

The Author

Jackie Pool

Jackie is an occupational therapist specialising in dementia care. She qualified in 1988 and, following her work as a clinical practitioner in the NHS and local authority, formed her own training and consultancy organisation in 1990. Jackie is an Alzheimer's Society approved trainer and has published several works on the care of older people with dementia, including books, journal articles, training manuals and chapters in textbooks. Jackie is also a regular speaker at national and international conferences on the subject of dementia care.

The Contributors

Sarah Mould

Sarah joined Jackie Pool Associates Ltd as Training and Development Consultant. She has been an occupational therapist for older people with mental health problems since 1994. Before this she worked as a clinician and manager within the NHS, with a lead for education, development and training for the older people's mental health directorate. Sarah is continually updating her knowledge and skills in the field of dementia care and is highly committed to the development of person-centred care services.

Jennifer Wenborn MSc DipCOT

Jennifer has worked as an occupational therapist for nearly 30 years, predominantly with older people. She has wide experience in hospital and community settings, providing physical and mental health services; as a clinician and manager; and has also worked as an independent practitioner. She is currently Clinical Research Fellow in Occupational Therapy at University College London. The PAL study was the first phase in her PhD research, a randomised controlled trial, 'Does occupational therapy intervention for people with dementia in a care home setting improve quality of life?'. Jennifer has written extensively about activity provision within care homes, including co-authoring *The Successful Activity Co-ordinator* (Hurtley and Wenborn, 2005, published by Age Concern).

Professor David Challis PhD

Professor of Community Care, Personal Social Services Research Unit, University of Manchester, UK

David Challis is Professor of Community Care Research and Director of the PSSRU at the University of Manchester. He is responsible for a series of evaluations of the effectiveness and efficiency of intensive care management for older people which have been influential in the development of community care services in the UK. He has also acted as an advisor on care management to a number of governments and service providers in the USA, Canada, Australia and Japan. Current areas of activity include a range of studies on assessment of older people and patterns of service provision. He has authored 19 books and editions, and written over 150 articles and chapters.

Professor Martin Orrell PhD FRCPsych

Professor of Ageing and Mental Health, University College London and North East London Mental Health Trust (NELMHT)

Martin trained at the Maudsley Hospital and the Institute of Psychiatry before being appointed at UCL in 1991. At NELMHT he works as an Honorary Consultant Old Age Psychiatrist, Associate Medical Director for Mental Health Services for Older People, and is Director of Research and Development. In recent years he has also worked as Specialist Advisor to the Health Advisory Service and Clinical Advisor to the Audit Commission for the 'Forget Me Not' national study on Mental Health Services for Older People. His research interests include needs assessment, health services evaluation, and psychosocial interventions for dementia, and he has published over 100 academic papers. He is Editor of the journal *Aging and Mental Health*, Course Director for MSc in Ageing and Mental Health at UCL, and Director of the London Centre for Dementia Care.

Preface

Since it was first published, the Pool Activity Level (PAL) Instrument has become the framework for activity-based care systems in a variety of settings for clients with cognitive impairments caused by conditions related to dementia, strokes and learning disabilities.

Following a validity and reliability research study of the PAL Checklist and recommendations in the National Clinical Practice Guideline for Dementia (NICE 2006), for use of the PAL Instrument for activity of daily living skills training and for activity planning, the author has added new material to the Guide. The content has been expanded to include statistical evidence from the research study. The newly developed second part of the Guide offers a selection of activities, with sources for obtaining them and guidance for carrying them out with individuals who have different levels of ability as revealed by the completion of the PAL Instrument Checklist. This third edition of the Guide gives new information about the statistical evidence for the reliability and validty of the PAL Checklist.

The Guide is designed to enable carers at home and in formal care settings to use the Pool Activity Level (PAL) Instrument to engage people with cognitive impairment in meaningful occupation. People with cognitive impairments may have difficulty engaging in activities, particularly if the activity is too demanding or not presented to the person in an understandable way. Care staff trying to provide leisure activity programmes can be at a loss to know how to offer the activity to maximise success, or how to find equipment locally or nationally.

Substantially revised, this edition continues to include the Instrument in photocopiable format of activity checklists and plans, which take into account users' life histories and help to match abilities with activities. You may wish to contact the author at enquiries@jackie-pool-associates.co.uk to source the photocopiable Instrument in electronic format so that you can print off the checklists, plans and outcome measures as you need them.

Guiding the reader through a series of clear, practical steps and using case studies to enable them to understand, plan and implement activities for clients, this is an essential resource for any practitioner or carer wanting to provide fulfilling occupation for clients with cognitive impairments.

To assist carers to facilitate leisure activities a further section has been added to this third edition of the PAL Instrument Guide. In Part 2 of this edition, ideas for four Activity Packs are set out in four chapters. A selection of possible activities, with sources for obtaining them and guidance for carrying them out with individuals who have different levels of ability as revealed by the completion of the PAL Instrument Checklist.

REFERENCE

National Institute for Health and Clinical Excellence (NICE) (2006) *Dementia: Supporting People with Dementia and Their Carers in Health and Social Care.* National Clinical Practice Guideline number 42. London: NICE, p.188.

Part 1 – The Pool Activity Level (PAL) Instrument

Chapter 1

Introduction to Part 1

USING THIS GUIDE

The PAL Instrument is based on the underpinning principle that people with cognitive impairment also have abilities and that when an enabling environment is presented to the person, these potential abilities can be realised. Occupation is the key to unlocking this potential. In order to present an occupation to the person with cognitive impairment so that he or she can engage with it, his or her impairments and abilities must first be understood. In addition, an individual is motivated to engage in occupations that have personal significance. Therefore an understanding of what drives the person, using information about his or her unique biography and about personality, is also vital. The PAL Instrument provides the user with the means to collect this important information and to use it to compile an individual profile that aids in the presentation of occupations to the person.

The PAL Instrument comprises:

- Life History Profile

- Checklist describing the way that an individual engages in occupations

- Activity Profile with general information for engaging the person in a range of meaningful occupation

- Individual Action Plan that includes directions for facilitating the engagement of the person in activities of daily living

- Outcome Sheet.

A blank copy of the PAL Instrument is in this Guide and may be photocopied for use by those working with people with cognitive impairment.

THEORETICAL BACKGROUND

The Pool Activity Level (PAL) Instrument draws from several models of understanding human behaviour: the Lifespan Approach to human development; the Dialectical Model of a person-centred approach to the interplay of social, neurological and psychological factors; and the Functional Information Processing Model.

The Lifespan Approach to human development

Theorists of human development propose that individuals' physical, intellectual, social and emotional skills change over time, according to the experiences they encounter. When this process is viewed in this way it is termed the Lifespan Approach. The first major theorist to acknowledge the lifelong nature of human development was Erik Erikson (Atkinson, Atkinson and Hilgard 1983) who described the 'Eight Ages of Man', each of which presents the individual with a new developmental activities to be worked on. Erikson proposed that human development does not end when physical maturity is reached, but that it is a continuous process from birth through to old age. His eight stages were based on the belief that the psychological development of an individual depends on the social relations he or she experiences at various points in life. When working with people with cognitive impairment it is helpful not only to recognise the importance of this cradle-to-grave development theory, but also to understand some of the developmental processes that take place in infancy and childhood. A more detailed description of developmental theory can be found elsewhere, but a brief description of neurological development is included here in order to clarify the theory underpinning the PAL Instrument.

When a child is born, the higher part of the brain is like a blank page waiting to be written on as experiences are encountered. The higher part of the brain is concerned with cognition, which includes functions such as thought, judgement, comprehension and reasoning. It also controls complex functions such as processing information from the environment sent from the sensory organs – the eyes, ears, nose, mouth and skin – via the nervous system to the brain. Infants learn from these experiences, which are 'written on' to the higher brain as memories in the form of patterns of nerve connections. This enables infants to judge new experiences against previous ones and to make decisions about how to respond. They also begin to be able to adapt to new situations as these arise by matching the experience to similar ones. It is a function of the higher brain to interpret information and to decide on the necessary action.

At first, the new-born baby is relying on the more primitive underlying part of the brain, which is concerned with basic emotions and needs. This primitive brain is responsible for early behaviour such as fear of strangers and the forming of a bond or specific attachment with another person. It also causes individuals, throughout their life, to experience and communicate social-emotional nuances (via emotional speech, laughing, crying, expressing sympathy, compassion) and to desire to form and maintain an emotional attachment. The primitive brain therefore enables us to be what is essentially a person: to establish the identity and existence that is conferred on us through contact with others.

The Dialectical Model of a person-centred approach

This model was proposed by Tom Kitwood when exploring factors other than neurological impairment that combine to cause the disability of dementia. One way of viewing these factors is as an equation where: $D = P + B + H + NI + SP$ (Kitwood 1993). This is a simple way of showing that any individual's dementia (D) is the result of a complex interaction between five main components: personality (P), biography (B), health (H), neurological impairment (NI) and social psychology (SP). To view dementia only as a result of the neurological impairment caused by the medical picture of Alzheimer's disease, for example, would be to view an incomplete picture. An individual's personality and life history will colour and shape the picture, although for the most part these will have been fully developed and are unchangeable.

Physical and mental ill health often cause people to behave differently as they try to cope with feelings of pain or discomfort. Some people with neurological impairments are unable to communicate their need to others verbally. Their behaviour, which is another form of communication, can be misinterpreted as part of their condition and the inappropriate response from others contributes further to the disability of the individual.

The final component of social psychology in the equation is viewed as the one that can have the most significant impact, either for better or worse. This is how the effects of meetings with others can impact on the emotional state of the person and either add to the disability of the person by undermining skills and causing feelings of ill-being, or reduce the disability by creating an environment that is empowering to the person and nurtures well-being.

A person-centred philosophy therefore recognises the uniqueness of the person more than his or her impairment. However, all of the factors that combine within the person need to be understood so that disability is minimised or avoided. Relationships are felt to be at the heart of person-centred philosophy and positive contacts with others can ensure the well-being of people with dementia, regardless of the level of impairment.

Well-being can be described as the state of having a sense of hope, agency, self-confidence and self-esteem. Hope in this way refers to a sense of expectation of positive experiences. Agency refers to a sense of having an impact on the surrounding environment and of being able to make things happen. Self-confidence refers to the feeling of assurance in one's own ability.

Self-esteem is a feeling of self-worth. The human need for occupation is satisfied when engagement in it also nurtures these states of well-being.

The Functional Information Processing Model

Cognition is the process by which we think and understand. When a person has a cognitive impairment, it may have one or more of several possible causes – illness, trauma, congenital differences, emotional stress – but in all cases there is damage to the nerve and brain tissue, most commonly in the higher brain. This damage causes cognitive impairments of judgement, reasoning, thinking and planning, which in turn can lead to disability such as dementia or learning disability. This will be the case if the physical and social environment is disempowering rather than compensating the person for the impairment or enabling him or her to adapt.

The Functional Information Processing Model is a model whose clinical application is grounded in occupational therapy (Pool 2006). Claudia K. Allen, an American occupational therapist, developed the model during her observations of clients with psychiatric disorders. The original theoretical base was influenced by Piaget's theory that cognitive development is a stage process (Piaget 1952). The cognitive model proposed by Piaget looks at the processes of human memory and puts great emphasis on aspects of being that require highly developed mental skills, but gives little consideration to feelings, emotions and relationships. Allen's later work (Allen 1999) has developed the theoretical base to include the work of Soviet psychologist Vygotsky, who proposed that human development is a social process involving close interactions between the child and its parents, and later its peers and teachers (Vygotsky 1978).

Allen's description of cognitive disability, based on these earlier theoretical bases, proposes that 'a restriction in voluntary motor action originating in the physical and chemical structures of the brain will produce observable limitations in routine task behaviour' (Allen 1985). Therefore, observing an individual's ability to carry out activities can indicate damage to those structures. This is because the cognitive processes driving the motor actions in order for the activities to be carried out are impaired.

Allen organised this evidence of cognitive impairment into six levels, using descriptions of how an individual attends to the environment, sensory cues and objects. These cognitive levels, which measure a person's ability to function, are based on the stages of development proposed by Piaget. By identifying the cognitive disability of an individual, occupational therapists can also identify his or her remaining abilities. The occupational therapist's role is then to design and test activity environments that utilise these abilities, and to instruct others in maintaining those environments.

The Pool Activity Level (PAL) Instrument takes the information from Allen's Functional Information Processing Model and presents it in a form that is accessible to those without an occupational therapy qualification. It provides the user with a self-interpreting assessment in the form of guides for creating and maintaining facilitating environments. The PAL further develops Allen's more recent attention to the importance of social connections in occupational performance, building on Vygotsky's insights into the importance of providing appropriate assistance and support to the individual while he or she engages in an activity. The PAL Instrument also combines the Functional Information Processing Model with the Socio-psychological Model by focusing the user on the biography of the individual and using this information as a guide to facilitating activities that are meaningful to him or her.

REFERENCES

Allen, C.K. (1985) *Occupational Therapy for Psychiatric Diseases: Measurement and Management of Cognitive Disabilities.* Boston: Little, Brown.

Allen, C.K. (1999) *Structures of the Cognitive Performance Modes.* Ormond Beach, Florida: Allen Conferences, Inc.

Atkinson, R.L., Atkinson, R.C. and Hilgard, E.R. (1983) *Introduction to Psychology* (International Edition). New York: Harcourt Brace Jonavich, pp.96–99.

Kitwood, T. (1993) 'Discover the Person, not the Disease.' *Journal of Dementia Care 1*, 1, 16–17.

Piaget, J. (1952) *The Origins of Intelligence in Children.* New York: International Universities Press, p.311.

Pool, J. (2006) 'The Functional Information Processing Model.' In E. Duncan (ed.) *Foundations for Practice in Occupational Therapy,* 4th edition. Edinburgh: Elsevier Churchill Livingstone.

Vygotsky, L.S. (1978) *The Development of Higher Psychological Processes.* Boston: Harvard University Press.

Chapter 2

The Four Activity Levels

Completing the Pool Activity Level (PAL) Checklist enables care givers to recognise the ability of a person with cognitive impairment to engage in activity. Any individual who knows the person well, by considering how he or she generally functions when carrying out activities (particularly those involving other people) can complete it. These observations should have been made in several situations over a period of two weeks. If the person lives in a group setting, such as a home, the observations may need to be a compilation from all involved care givers. In this way the variation of abilities and disabilities that can occur in an individual over a period of time is taken into account, and an Occupational Profile can be made. The Occupational Profile gives an overview of the way in which a person best engages in activities and how to create a facilitating environment.

Because there are many factors affecting an individual's ability to engage in an activity – cognitive integrity, the meaningfulness of the activities, the familiarity of the environment, the support of others – it is likely that an individual will reveal a variation in his or her level of ability in different activities. The PAL Instrument acknowledges the importance of this and provides the opportunity to create an Individual Action Plan that allows for a varying degree of support in some of the personal activities of daily living.

The PAL is organised into four activity levels: planned, exploratory, sensory and reflex.

PLANNED ACTIVITY LEVEL

At a planned activity level the person can work towards completing activities but may not be able to solve any problems that arise while in the process. He or she will be able to look in obvious places for equipment needed but may not be able to search beyond the usual places. A care giver assisting someone at this level will need to keep his or her sentences short and avoid using words like 'and' or 'but' which tend to be used to link two sentences together into a more complex one. Care givers will also need to stand by to help solve any problems should they arise. People functioning at a planned activity level are able to carry out activities that achieve a tangible result.

EXPLORATORY ACTIVITY LEVEL

At an exploratory activity level the person can carry out very familiar activities in familiar surroundings. However, at this level people are more concerned with the effect of carrying out the activity than in the consequence and may not have an end result in mind. Therefore a creative and spontaneous approach by care givers to activities is helpful. If an activity involves more than two or three activities, a person at this level will need help in breaking the activity into manageable chunks. Directions need to be made very simple and the use of memory aids such as activities lists, calendars and labelling of frequently used items can be very helpful.

SENSORY ACTIVITY LEVEL

At a sensory activity level the person may not have many thoughts or ideas about carrying out an activity; he or she is mainly concerned with sensation and with moving his or her body in response to those sensations. People at this level can be guided to carry out single-step activities such as sweeping or winding wool. More complex activities can only be carried out when directed one step at a time. Therefore care givers need to ensure that the person at this activity level has the opportunity to experience a wide variety of sensations and to carry out one-step activities. Directions to maximise this opportunity need to be kept very simple and to be reinforced by demonstrating the action required.

REFLEX ACTIVITY LEVEL

A person at a reflex activity level may not be aware of the surrounding environment or even of his or her own body. He or she is living in a subliminal or subconscious state where movement is a reflex response to a stimulus. Therefore people wishing to enter into this person's consciousness need to use direct sensory stimulation. By using direct stimulation the person's self-awareness can be raised. A person at this level may have difficulty in organising more than one sensation which is being experienced at the same time. Excessive or multiple stimuli can cause distress; therefore crowds, loud noises and background clamour should be avoided. Activities at this level should focus on introducing a single sensation to the person. A care giver interacting with a person at a reflex level needs to use all his or her communication skills to enter into the world of a person at this level. Language skills tend to play only a minor role at this level and should be kept to single-word directions, although the use of facial expression and of a warm and reassuring tone and appropriate volume can be vital in establishing a communication channel.

Chapter 3

Reliability and Validity of the PAL Checklist

Jennifer Wenborn, David Challis and Martin Orrell

INTRODUCTION

Development of the PAL Instrument is outlined in the Introduction to Part 1 of this Guide. It is now used in a variety of service settings for older people with dementia care throughout the UK and beyond. General opinion obtained through professional networks suggested that it is a useful and practical tool. Indeed, it is recommended in the National Clinical Practice Guideline for Dementia (NICE 2006) as an instrument to guide providers of daily living and leisure activities. This acknowledges that, in order for care staff to integrate occupational opportunities into their daily care provision, they need a quick and easy-to-use assessment tool. Assessment tools do need to be 'fit for purpose', and this can be demonstrated by assessing their psychometric properties (the technical construction and qualities of the instrument) (Bowling 2002), to ensure they are valid and reliable for use, both in practice and research.

AIM OF THE STUDY

The aim of this study was to assess the validity and reliability of the PAL Checklist when used with older people who have dementia.

METHOD

Study design

There were two phases to the study. Phase One used a postal questionnaire to assess content validity. Phase Two assessed the criterion, concurrent and construct validity; internal consistency; and inter-rater and test-retest reliability in a sample of older people with dementia.

Validity

Validity refers to how well an instrument assesses the concept that it is intended to assess (Bowling 2002). In this case, the concept is the individual's cognitive level of ability to engage in activity. Several aspects of validity can be measured. Content validity considers the extent to which the instrument assesses the scope of the concept. It is commonly measured by consulting experts in the field and professionals, users and carers relevant to the area.

Other aspects of validity, such as criterion, concurrent and construct validity, can be measured by comparing the performance of the instrument, alongside other relevant assessments, with a group of participants from the target population – in this case, older people with dementia.

Reliability

Reliability considers how consistent the instrument is (Bowling 2002). There are three aspects. *Internal consistency* refers to how the results obtained for each test item correlate with each other. *Inter-rater reliability* refers to the test's consistency when used by different assessors. *Test-retest reliability* looks at how far the results are consistent when the test is repeated (for example, a week later). Assuming the clinical picture has not changed then if the test is reliable the results would be very similar.

Phase One – Content validity

A postal questionnaire was sent to three groups:

1.   the College of Occupational Therapists Specialist Section – Older People's Dementia Clinical Forum

2.   The National Association for Providers of Activities for Older People (NAPA) and

3.   other experts, mainly occupational therapists and activity providers.

The questionnaire asked respondents to indicate their professional background using the following options: occupational therapist (OT); occupational therapy assistant/technician; activity provider; care assistant; nurse; doctor; psychologist;

social worker; other (please specify). Respondents were asked if they had previously used the PAL Checklist and, if so, in what type of setting: ward/day service/person's home/care home? The following questions were asked: 'Are any important items missing?'; 'Are any items redundant?'; 'Are the instructions clear?' Each of these questions required the respondent to circle either 'yes' or 'no' and space for further comment or explanation was provided. Finally, respondents were asked, 'How easy or difficult do you think it is to complete the PAL Checklist?' and given four options to choose from: very difficult, quite difficult, quite easy, very easy. Finally, respondents were asked to rank the importance of each of the nine Checklist items using a four-point scale, when 1 = not important; 2 = quite important; 3 = very important; and 4 = essential. The number of responses to each item in the questionnaire was counted, and the percentages calculated for each category.

Phase Two – Validity and reliability

A sample of 60 older people with dementia was recruited from a range of in-patient, day hospital and continuing care services provided within a NHS mental health trust. Participants had to: be aged 60 years or over; have received the service for at least two weeks (or four visits in the case of day hospitals); meet the criteria often used to diagnose dementia (American Psychiatric Association 1994); and score less than 24 on the Mini Mental State Examination (MMSE) (Folstein, Folstein and McHugh 1975). Information sheets explaining the study were provided and, if possible, consent was obtained directly from participants. For those people who were not able to sign a consent form, their potential participation was discussed with their relatives (if applicable) and/or a relevant member of staff (for example, their key worker) in order to protect their best interests. Participants' general practitioners were informed that they were taking part in the study. The NHS Barking and Havering Local Research Ethics Committee provided ethical approval (reference number: 05/Q0602/8).

INSTRUMENTS

The Pool Activity Level (PAL) Checklist (Pool 2002)

Please see Chapter 9 for a complete PAL Instrument including the Checklist. The following package of instruments was also used in the study.

Mini Mental State Examination (MMSE) (Folstein *et al.* 1975)

The MMSE is a well-known cognitive screening test frequently used in clinical and research settings. Validity, test-retest and inter-rater reliability were established by the original authors (Folstein *et al.* 1975) and have been further reviewed by Tombaugh and McIntyre (1992). The maximum score of 30 indicates no cognitive impairment. It was predicted that higher MMSE scores would correlate with higher PAL activity levels.

Clinical Dementia Rating Scale (CDR) (Hughes *et al.* 1982)

The CDR is a global rating of the severity of dementia. Inter-rater reliability has been established (Berg *et al.* 1988; Hughes *et al.* 1982). The Chronic Care Version includes two further categories of severity: profound and terminal. It was therefore used in this study to cover the range of service settings included. The lowest possible score of 0 indicates no evidence of dementia and a score of 5 indicates the most severe level. It was predicted that lower CDR scores would correlate with higher PAL activity levels.

Barthel Index (BI) (Mahoney and Barthel 1965)

The BI measures functional ability and the degree of assistance required (physical and/or verbal) in ten daily living activities. The score indicates the individual's level of dependency. Validity, inter-rater and test-retest reliability and sensitivity have been assessed as being excellent (Wade and Collin 1988). The activities assessed by both the BI and the PAL Checklist are: bathing/washing, getting dressed, eating. The maximum score of 100 indicates independence in daily living activities. It was predicted that higher BI scores would correlate with higher PAL activity levels.

Bristol Activities of Daily Living Scale (BADLS) (Bucks *et al.* 1996)

The BADLS is a carer-rated scale comprising 20 items. It was developed specifically for use with people with dementia. Face, construct and concurrent validity, and test-retest reliability have been confirmed (Bucks *et al.* 1996). The activities assessed by both the BADLS and the PAL Checklist are: bathing/washing, dressing, eating, communication and participation in activities. The lowest possible score of 0 indicates independence in daily living activities, while the highest possible score of 60 indicates maximum dependence. It was predicted that lower BADLS scores would correlate with higher PAL activity levels.

Clifton Assessment Procedures for the Elderly – Behaviour Rating Scale (CAPE-BRS) (Pattie and Gilleard 1979)

The CAPE-BRS is a carer-rated scale that assesses a range of daily living activities and behaviours, with the aim of indicating the individual's level of dependency. Four subsections consider: physical dependency, apathy, communication difficulties, and social disturbance. The activities assessed by both the CAPE-BRS and the PAL Checklist are: bathing, dressing, participation in activity, socialising, and communication. The lowest possible score of 0 indicates independent function, while the highest possible score of 36 indicates maximum dependency. It was predicted that lower CAPE-BRS scores would correlate with higher PAL activity levels.

Assessing validity

Three raters, all occupational therapists working within the NHS trust, collected the data using the following process. The MMSE was completed with the participant with dementia. A member of staff was interviewed about each participant and asked to complete the PAL Checklist. Their observations of how the individual had actually behaved over the previous two weeks, plus information obtained from the individual's care plan, enabled the rater to complete the other instruments: CDR, BI, BADLS, CAPE-BRS.

Criterion validity was assessed by comparing the PAL activity levels by service setting. It had been predicted that the participants who were attending a day hospital, i.e. they were still living in the community, would achieve a higher PAL activity level than those living in continuing care.

Construct validity was evaluated using an inter-item correlation matrix. It had been anticipated that the highest correlation would be within two groups of activities. The first group comprised: bathing/washing, getting dressed, practical activities, use of objects and looking at a newspaper/magazine; as these all rely on being able to recognise and use objects appropriately and in the correct sequence. The second group comprised: contact with others, groupwork skills and communication skills; as these all depend on interacting and communicating with other people.

Concurrent validity was measured by correlating the PAL Checklist results with the test scores obtained using the other instruments. There is no relevant 'gold standard' instrument against which to directly compare the PAL Checklist, i.e. a generic, quick and easy-to-use tool that assesses an individual's level of ability to engage in activities. The other instruments were therefore selected because they either assess: key factors that influence the ability to engage in activity, such as the severity of dementia (CDR) and degree of cognitive impairment (MMSE); or the ability to carry out specific activities that are also assessed by the PAL Checklist (BI, BADLS, CAPE-BRS).

Assessing reliability

Inter-rater reliability was measured by asking a second member of staff to complete the PAL Checklist on the same day, without discussing or comparing the results. Test-retest reliability was measured by asking the same member of staff to complete the PAL Checklist again about a week later.

RESULTS

Phase One

A total of 122 questionnaires were circulated and 102 completed questionnaires were received, which represents a response rate of 84 per cent. Fifty-five (54%) respondents had previously used the PAL Checklist and 47 (46%) had not. Of those who had used the instrument, 25 (45%) had used it in a ward; 20 (36%) in a day service; 22 (40%) in a person's own home; and 27 (49%) in a care-home setting. Seventy-five (74%) were occupational therapists or occupational therapy support workers; 12 (12%) were activity providers; and the other 14 (14%) were from a variety of professional backgrounds, including nursing and psychology.

Content validity

Ninety-five (97%) said the instructions for completing the PAL Checklist were clear. Using a four-point scale ranging from 'very difficult' to 'very easy', 90 respondents (93%) rated the PAL Checklist as 'quite easy' or 'very easy' to complete. Seven items were ranked as very important or essential by at least 73 (77%) of respondents. The most highly ranked of these seven items was contact with others, by 93 (99%) of respondents. This was followed by: communication skills, 89 (94%); eating, 87 (93%); getting dressed, 79 (84%); bathing/washing, 78 (82%); use of objects, 74 (78%); and practical activities, 73 (77%). Fifty-seven (60%) ranked groupwork skills as very important or essential, and a further 33 (35%) ranked it as quite important. Only 30 (32%) respondents ranked the newspaper item as very important or essential, but a further 45 (47%) ranked it as quite important. Most respondents (48 or 55%) said no important items were missing, although 39 (45%) said that one or more important items were missing, and 52 (60%) made comments that there was no consistent pattern to their responses. Nine (17%) responses related to describing the individual's mood and motivation, for example: 'perhaps "mood" or "ability to co-operate" could be included?' Eight (15%) commented on the individual's level of orientation and/or ability to navigate their environment, for example: 'orientation to place, e.g. ability to find way around familiar/unfamiliar buildings or places'. Five (10%) responses suggested the inclusion of mobility and another five (10%) felt that 'having information and assessment of a person's ability to transfer, i.e. on and off bed, chair and toilet' was needed. A further five (10%) specifically suggested that using the toilet and/or continence should be included.

Twenty-four (27%) respondents felt that there were some redundant items. Their comments related mainly to two items, 'groupwork skills' (13 or 15%) and 'looking at a newspaper/magazine' (14 or 16%), and were based on the practitioners' own experience of using the instrument. The difficulty of completing the groupwork skills item when assessing people living on their own in the community was highlighted. Its relevance was also questioned, as this approach is not seen as appropriate for those in the later stages of dementia. It was also pointed out that 'groupwork is the kind of skill which has something to do with staff'. There were three themes related to the newspaper item: some felt it can be difficult to assess; others that it may not be a familiar activity to some people, and therefore not relevant to assess; while others stated, 'it is very specific', suggesting that 'this may be better widened to include other similar activities, e.g. TV'.

Phase Two

Data were collected for 60 people with dementia. There were 20 from each of the following service settings: day hospital, in-patient ward, and continuing care. Twenty-five (42%) participants were male and thrity-five (58%) were female. The participants' ages ranged from 64 to 96, with a mean (average) age of 78 years. Twenty (33%) lived in continuing care. The social situation of the remaining 40 people, when not in hospital, was as follows: 16 (40%) lived alone; 18 (45%) lived with a spouse or relative; and six (15%) lived in supported accommodation. The MMSE scores ranged from 0 to 22, with a mean score of 9. Fifty-five staff were interviewed to enable completion of the instruments. Their length of experience working with older people with dementia ranged from 10 months to 27 years. Twenty-eight (51%) had a professional qualification (primarily registered mental nurse). Twelve (22%) had an NVQ or equivalent level qualification and the other 15 (27%) had no formal qualification.

Criterion validity

The frequency of the PAL activity levels and each Checklist item within each of the service settings is shown in Table 3.1. The frequency of PAL activity levels for the total sample (60) was 18 (30%) at planned level, 11 (18%) at exploratory level, 12 (20%) at sensory level and 19 (32%) at reflex level. Table 3.1 demonstrates that, as predicted, the day-hospital attendees achieved higher PAL activity levels, which indicates a higher level of ability than those requiring the additional support provided within a continuing care setting. Conversely, those in continuing care obtained lower PAL activity levels, thus reflecting their higher level of dependency.

**Table 3.1 Frequency (%) of PAL activity levels
and PAL Checklist items per service setting (n = 60)**

PAL activity level	Day hospital	In-patient	Continuing care
Planned	11 (55%)	4 (20%)	3 (15%)
Exploratory	3 (15%)	5 (25%)	3 (15%)
Sensory	5 (25%)	7 (35%)	0 (0%)
Reflex	1 (5%)	4 (20%)	14 (70%)

Concurrent validity

Concurrent validity was demonstrated through correlating the PAL Checklist scores with scores on the other instruments, using Spearman's rank order correlation coefficient (rho). The rho value for each correlation was as follows: MMSE (-0.75); BI (-0.71); CAPE-BRS (0.71); BADLS (0.82); and CDR (0.81). A minimum value of 0.7 is recommended and the nearer the value is to 1.0, the stronger is the correlation. All correlations were therefore highly significant ($p < 0.001$). As expected, the (negative) correlation with the MMSE and BI reflected that higher scores obtained using these tools indicate higher levels of cognitive ability and independence in daily living activities respectively and therefore correlate with higher PAL activity levels. Conversely, the (positive) correlation with the CAPE-BRS, BADLS and CDR reflect that higher scores obtained using these tools indicate: higher dependency; poorer ability to perform daily living activities; and more severe dementia respectively; and so correlate with lower PAL activity levels.

Construct validity

The correlation between each item of the PAL Checklist is shown in Table 3.2. In terms of convergent validity, again using Spearman's rank order correlation coefficient (rho), the highest correlations were found between practical activities and use of objects (0.81); getting dressed (0.80) and bathing/washing (0.79); and between the newspaper item and use of objects (0.76). High correlation was also found between contact with others and groupwork skills (0.77).

Table 3.2 Construct validity: inter-item correlation of the PAL Checklist

	Getting dressed	Eating	Contact with others	Groupwork skills	Communication skills	Practical activities	Use of objects	Newspaper
Bathing	0.76	0.59	0.65	0.65	0.72	0.79	0.71	0.70
Dressing		0.63	0.63	0.76	0.71	0.80	0.79	0.63
Eating			0.56	0.53	0.75	0.65	0.69	0.60
Contact				0.77	0.72	0.56	0.64	0.68
Groupwork					0.68	0.69	0.67	0.70
Communica-tion						0.75	0.80	0.74
Practical							0.81	0.74
Use of objects								0.76

Spearman's rank order correlation (rho) used

Internal consistency

The Cronbach's alpha coefficient value was 0.95. This statistical test measures the average correlation of all the test items. A minimum value of 0.7 is recommended, and the nearer the value is to 1.0, then the stronger the reliability. This therefore indicates that the scale had excellent internal consistency.

Inter-rater and test-retest reliability

Reliability was measured using two statistical tests: Cohen's Kappa and the intra class coefficient (ICC). Initially the maximum range of all four activity levels was analysed using a 4 x 4 table. However, because the full range of levels was not used for one item (eating), the ICC values could not be calculated. The data was therefore recoded and analysed, by combining the planned and exploratory level results together, and combining the sensory and reflex level results together. This reflected the natural division observed within the data, as well as clinical experience of using the PAL Checklist. The Kappa and ICC values for inter-rater and test-retest reliability are summarised in Table 3.3. Various 'yardsticks' can be used to define these values, but the following is commonly used: a Kappa value less than 0.40 indicates poor agreement; 0.40 to 0.59 is fair; 0.60 to 0.74 is good; and 0.75 to 1.00 indicates excellent agreement; and an ICC of 0.80 and above indicates that the scale is highly reliable (Bowling 2002). Using these values, all items achieved fair, good or excellent inter-rater and test-retest reliability.

DISCUSSION

This study showed that the PAL Checklist has adequate validity and reliability, and, as such, provides a robust psychometric underpinning for its widespread use in clinical practice. It suggests it will also be useful in research with people who have dementia. The questionnaire response rate was excellent. This could be said to indicate the respondents' level of interest in establishing validated tools for use in this setting. The instructions for completion were rated as clear and the Checklist was seen as reasonably easy to complete. This reflects the previous anecdotal feedback from practitioners. It would therefore appear to fulfil the original design remit, which was to produce a practical resource for care staff working with people with dementia to enable their engagement in meaningful activities.

Content validity was strong with most respondents stating that no important items were missing. There was no consistent pattern of response from those

Table 3.3 Reliability: Kappa and intra-class coefficient values (ICC)

	Inter-rater Kappa	ICC	Test-retest Kappa	ICC
PAL level	0.54	0.69	0.76	0.87
Bathing/washing	0.53	0.61	0.70	0.81
Getting dressed	0.56	0.77	0.76	0.84
Eating	0.94	0.93	1.0	0.96
Contact with others	0.46	0.62	0.57	0.77
Groupwork skills	0.42	0.62	0.58	0.78
Communication skills	0.63	0.72	0.76	0.84
Practical activities	0.66	0.70	0.75	0.86
Use of objects	0.43	0.63	0.55	0.72
Looking at a newspaper/magazine	0.57	0.62	0.65	0.75

suggesting additional items for inclusion. Mood and motivation was suggested as an additional item, but while this is obviously an important factor in selecting and presenting activity, it would not be appropriate to include in a scale that assesses cognitive ability to engage in an activity. Another suggestion was the inclusion of orientation and ability to navigate the environment. However, while this depends in part on cognitive components, it is also greatly influenced by the environment itself and how familiar and/or well designed it is. Lastly, the suggestion to include further daily living activities perhaps reflects the common emphasis on personal care rather than other activities and the tendency observed in some practice settings to use the PAL Checklist as an assessment of daily living activities, which it is not designed to be.

The comments regarding redundant items reflect the first author's clinical experience that care staff in continuing care settings often find the groupwork skills difficult to assess; and that staff in all three settings frequently find the newspaper item difficult to assess as newspapers and magazines are not always routinely available. These comments were also reflected in the ranking of the importance of each item, with the newspaper and groupwork skills items being scored as very important or essential by 32 per cent and 60 per cent of the respondents respectively. This is a much lower percentage than that given to the other seven items, which were rated at the higher level of importance by more than three quarters of the respondents.

The frequency of the PAL activity levels and responses for each of the Checklist items within each of the service settings mainly confirmed clinical experience and expectations. However, the absence of anyone being assessed at the sensory level within the continuing care settings was surprising and contrasts with the clinical experience of the first author, a specialist practitioner within this area. Perhaps it reflects the difficulty of care staff in differentiating between the PAL activity levels when dealing with people who have more severe dementia, and indeed the tendency to underestimate a person's ability to engage. If so, it appears to reinforce Perrin's (1997, p.938) assertion that 'marked occupational poverty exists' for people with severe dementia.

The results for criterion validity were as predicted, with those people still living in the community achieving higher PAL activity levels. This reflects the relative levels of support and assistance (physical and/or verbal) that people with dementia in different care settings require to carry out activities. In practice, this information can be used to inform and thereby enable care givers to provide the appropriate level of support to the person, thus moving towards a more optimal balance between providing necessary assistance while also maintaining the individual's remaining abilities and level of independence.

Concurrent validity was high, demonstrating the relevance of taking the level of cognition and severity of dementia into consideration when selecting activities. The importance of using personal history information in combination with the Checklist results was highlighted by several respondents. This enables personally meaningful activities to be selected and then presented at the individual's level of ability.

Construct validity was also strong, with the predicted correlation of bathing/washing, getting dressed, practical activities, use of objects and looking at a newspaper/magazine being proven. The strongest correlations were observed between practical activities and the other items, save for the newspaper item, and as such bears out the clinical expectations. The absence of the newspaper item perhaps reflects the earlier comments reported under content validity. The high correlation between the newspaper item and use of objects supports Pool's original rationale when developing the tool, which included the newspaper item as a way of double-checking the ability to handle objects (Pool 2005). The other high correlation between contact with others and groupwork skills was also anticipated.

The overall reliability of the PAL Checklist was acceptable. The Cronbach's alpha value indicated excellent internal consistency. This highlights the contribution of each of the items when assessing the ability to engage in an activity. Inter-rater reliability was assessed as being fair, with individual items ranging from excellent to fair. The range of values for individual test items perhaps reflects variations in the role of the assessor and the particular service setting. For example, the staff in a day hospital who did not routinely provide personal care assistance found it difficult to assess the bathing/washing and getting dressed items. Staff were interviewed separately and asked not to confer. This reduced the risk of bias and thereby provided a more rigorous test of reliability. Bearing in mind the number of staff involved in the study, and their differing levels of qualification and experience, the fact that inter-rater reliability for each item was at least fair reflects how quick and easy it is to learn and put into practice with reasonable consistency. Test-retest reliability was assessed as being excellent. This would be expected for a tool that needs to be completed by care givers who know the person well, measuring a level of performance that would not be expected to change significantly over the course of a week or so. It may therefore be concluded that the PAL Checklist tool demonstrates adequate validity and reliability when used with older people with dementia, and it is also brief, clear and easy to use, and as such can be described as being fit for purpose.

REFERENCES

American Psychiatric Association (1994) *Diagnosis and Statistical Manual of Mental Disorders*, 4th edition. Washington DC: American Psychiatric Association.

Berg, L., Miller, J.P., Storandt, M. (1988) 'Mild Service Dementia of the Alzheimer Type: 2 Longitudinal Assessment.' *Annals of Neurology 23*, 477–84.

Bowling, A. (2002) *Research Methods in Health: Investigating Health and Health Services*, 2nd edition. Maidenhead: Open University, pp. 147–153.

Bucks, R.S., Ashworth, D.L., Wilcock, G.K. and Siegfried, K. (1996) 'Assessment of Activities of Daily Living in Dementia: Development of the Bristol Activities of Daily Living Scale.' *Age and Ageing 25*, 113–20.

Folstein, M.F., Folstein, S.E. and McHugh, P.R. (1975) 'Mini Mental State: A Practical Guide for Grading the Cognitive State of Patients for the Clinician.' *Journal of Psychiatric Research 12*, 3, 189–198.

Hughes, C.P., Berg, L., Daniziger, W.L., Coben, L.A. and Martin, R.L. (1982) 'A New Clinical Scale for the Staging of Dementia.' *British Journal of Psychiatry 140*, 566–572.

Mahoney, F.I. and Barthel, D.W. (1965) 'Functional Evaluation: The Barthel Index.' *Maryland State Medical Journal 14*, 61–65.

National Institute for Health and Clinical Excellence (NICE) (2006) *Dementia: Supporting People with Dementia and Their Carers in Health and Social Care*. National Clinical Practice Guideline number 42. London: NICE, p.188.

Pattie, A.H. and Gilleard, C.J. (1979) *Manual of the Clifton Assessment Procedures for the Elderly (CAPE)*. Sevenoaks: Hodder & Stoughton Educational.

Perrin, T. (1997) 'Occupational Need in Severe Dementia: A Descriptive Study.' *Journal of Advanced Nursing 25*, 934–941.

Pool, J. (2002) *The Pool Activity Level (PAL) Instrument for Occupational Profiling*. London: Jessica Kingsley Publishers.

Pool, J. (2005) Personal communication.

Tombaugh, T.N. and McIntyre, N.J. (1992) 'The Mini-Mental State Examination: A Comprehensive Review.' *Journal of the American Geriatrics Society 40*, 922–935.

Wade, D.T. and Collin, C. (1988) 'The Barthel ADL Index: A Standard Measure of Physical Disability?' *International Disability Studies 10*, 64–67.

ACKNOWLEDGEMENTS

JW would like to thank all the older people and her colleagues within North East London Mental Health NHS Trust (NELMHT) who contributed to this study, in particular her two co-raters, Jane Burgess and Nicola Elliott, Advanced Practitioner Occupational Therapists. She would also like to acknowledge: the funding of her post by the NELMHT Occupational Therapy Service; continued support of the NELMHT Research and Development Directorate; and the College of Occupational Therapists and the Hospital Savings Association (HSA) for the 2005 PhD Scholarship Award.

This chapter is based on a paper which was originally published as: Wenborn, J., Challis, D., Pool, J., Burgess, J. *et al.* (2007) 'Assessing the Validity and Reliability of the Pool Activity Level (PAL) Checklist for Use with Older People with Dementia.' We are grateful to the publisher of *Aging and Mental Health*, Taylor and Francis Group, Abingdon, UK, for permission to reprint some of the content here, with the appropriate contextual alterations.

Chapter 4

Life History Work

THE IMPORTANCE OF GATHERING A LIFE HISTORY

Life history or story work is recognised as an important process that should become a major influence in care planning as a means of 'engaging and interacting with people, in order to encourage and assist them to recall and record in tangible form their personal histories' (Gibson 2005, pp.175–179).

Life history differs from life review in that it does not require an evaluation of the information that is gathered. Whereas life review is a therapeutic approach to resolving past problems, life history work is not directly aimed at changing a person's view of himself or herself, but rather at care givers who are encouraged to recognise the whole person in the context of their lifespan. The factual account of an individual's life history builds up a full picture of the person. This perspective should assist care givers in their interactions with the person and in planning activities that relate to the person's interests and experiences. The result of this individualised care plan is to recognise the uniqueness of the person and to potentially make a significant change in the quality of his or her life. The purpose of a Personal History Profile is to enable carers to recognise the person as a unique individual and not to see only the person's disability.

The PAL Instrument Personal History Profile is a method that uses subheadings to guide the user when gathering relevant information. By finding out about all that the person has experienced it is possible to have a better understanding of the person's behaviour now. It also gives care workers, who may not know the person so well, topics of conversation that will have meaning for the person.

Putting together the Profile should be an enjoyable project that the person with cognitive impairment, relatives and care workers can join together in, encouraging social interaction and reminiscence. The information gained from the Personal History Profile informs the PAL Activity Profile by guiding activity selection.

GUIDELINES FOR GATHERING LIFE HISTORY INFORMATION USING THE POOL ACTIVITY LEVEL (PAL) PERSONAL HISTORY PROFILE

The questions in the Profile are very general, designed to cater for all people regardless of age or sex. Some questions may be irrelevant, and these should be ignored. If the person is being cared for in a home or hospital or is attending a day centre, it may be possible to ask family members to complete the whole form with the person at home. For others, completion of the Profile may be spread out over a period of weeks, as more information is revealed. The Profile is therefore not an assessment but a means of recording useful information in a systematic way.

Any photographs that are available can be added to the Profile. It is helpful to write on the reverse: the person's name; who is in the photograph; and where and when it was taken. Some relatives may be worried about the photographs getting lost or damaged. In these cases, the photographs can be photocopied, and the originals kept safe.

A sample of a completed Profile is included for information.

REFERENCE

Gibson, F. (2005) 'Fit for Life: The Contribution of Life Story Work.' In M. Marshall (ed.) *Perspectives on Rehabilitation and Dementia.* London: Jessica Kingsley Publishers.

Pool Activity Level (PAL) Personal History Profile

What Is Your Name?

Elsie Jones

When Were You Born?

10 November 1926

Childhood

Where were you born?	*Leeds, West Riding of Yorkshire*
What are your family members' names?	*Thomas and Molly Charlton (parents) Harry (older brother)*
What were your family members' occupations?	*Sweet shop owners (parents) Tram driver (Harry) but killed in Second World War*
Where did you live?	*Headingley, Leeds*
Which schools did you attend?	*Leeds Girls School*
What was your favourite subject?	*English and Sewing*
Did you have any family pets? What were their names?	*Cats: Charlie/Smudge*

Adolescence

When did you leave school?	*Age 14*
Where did you work?	*Parents' shop, then went to clothing factory, then opened own shop in York in 1952*
What did you do at work?	*Machinist at factory then owned dress shop*
Did you have any special training?	*Can't remember*
What special memories do you have of work days?	*Day trips in summer. Friend, Mary, machined across her finger*
Did you do National Service?	*No*

Adulthood

Do/did you have a partner?	Yes
Partner's name/occupation?	Sidney, bank clerk
Where and when did you meet?	At a dance in Leeds
Where and when did you marry?	5 May 1946 at Headingley Church
What did you wear? What flowers did you have?	Cream dress and roses
Where did you go on honey-moon?	Scarborough
Where did you live?	Leeds, moved to York when Sidney promoted
Any children – what are their names?	Shirley, March 1947
Any grandchildren – what are their names?	Susan, 1967 and Michael, 1969
Did you have any special friends?	Yes
What are their names?	Barbara
When and where did you meet? Are you still in touch?	Factory, see each other sometimes
Did you have any pets? What were their names?	Cats, latest one Susie is 19 years old

Retirement

When did you retire?	1986 age 60. Sidney retired from bank 1991
What were you looking forward to most?	Gardening together, touring, visiting family
What were your hobbies and interests?	Used to sew and read a lot but stopped when eyes got bad
What were the biggest changes for you?	Shirley moving away to London when she married

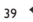

Likes and dislikes

What do you enjoy doing now?	*Like to listen to big band music, and to story tapes. Quizzes on the television*
What do you like to read?	*Thrillers, Agatha Christie*
What is your favourite colour?	*Yellow*
What kind of music do you like?	*Big band, Nat King Cole*
What are your favourite foods and drinks?	*Roast meals, chocolate, sherry*
Is there anything that you definitely do not like to do?	*Bingo*

How you like to do things

Do you have any special routines to your day?	*Main meal at lunch time, bath before bed and hot chocolate in bed to settle me*
What time do you like to get up in the morning? And go to bed at night?	*Get up at 9, go to bed after 10 o'clock news*
Do you want people to help you with anything?	*Doing up fastenings and getting in and out of the bath*
Do you want people to leave you to do anything on your own?	*Having a bath, getting dressed except for fastenings*
How do you like people to address you?	*Elsie*
What are you good at?	*Quizzes*
Is there anything else you would like to tell us about you?	*No*

Chapter 5

PAL Checklist Case Studies

Case Study 1

John is a retired school headmaster who lives with his wife. He is a very precise man who enjoys propagating plants and stamp collecting. Six months ago John went to his GP because he was worried about his increasingly poor memory. The GP diagnosed Alzheimer's disease. This is affecting John's ability to remember the names of friends, plants and stamps in his collection and he finds this frustrating and embarrassing. His wife is worried that this will lower John's confidence when out and will affect their weekly outings to local restaurants. Although he is able to select cutlery appropriately, he has become less socially outgoing and does not chat to the waiters as he used to.

Although John does have memory problems and is now not paying so much attention to the finer details and finishing touches in his hobbies, he still enjoys being involved in his hobbies with his wife's help.

When John is at ease with others, he is able to start conversations and enjoys discussing topics that he has noticed in the newspaper. Only people close to him realise that he has any disability, and only last week John enjoyed an afternoon with two close friends when they all successfully constructed and painted a new garden shed. There was one moment when he had difficulty with aligning the hinges on the door and could not solve the problem, but one of the others stepped in to help and John was able to carry on with another part of the project.

John is also able to use his own initiative to carry out most everyday activities. Although his wife has to remind him to have a wash and to shave, John is able to choose what to wear and to get dressed independently.

John and his wife are keen to plan ways of continuing his independence for as long as possible. When the Pool Activity Level (PAL) Checklist is completed for John it reveals that he is able to carry out activities at a planned level. It is now possible to use this information to help John to use his remaining abilities and to compensate for his disabilities.

Pool Activity Level (PAL) Checklist

Name: Date: Outcome:

John Porter   **1 September 2007**   **Planned**

Completing the Checklist: for each activity the statements refer to a different level of ability. Thinking of the last two weeks, tick the statement that represents the person's ability in each activity. There should be only one tick for each activity. If in doubt about which statement to tick, choose the level of ability that represents their average performance over the last two weeks. Make sure you tick one statement for each of the activities.

1. Bathing/Washing

- Can bathe/wash independently, sometimes with a little help to start   P: ☑

- Needs soap put on flannel and one-step-at-a-time directions to wash   E: ☐

- Mainly relies on others but will wipe own face and hands if encouraged   S: ☐

- Totally dependent and needs full assistance to wash or bathe   R: ☐

2. Getting dressed

- Plans what to wear, selects own clothing from cupboards; dresses in correct order   P: ☑

- Needs help to plan what to wear but recognises items and how to wear them; needs help with order of dressing   E: ☐

- Needs help to plan and with order of dressing, but can carry out small activities if someone directs each step   S: ☐

- Totally dependent on someone to plan, sequence and complete dressing; may move limbs to assist   R: ☐

3. Eating

- Eats independently and appropriately using the correct cutlery   P: ☑

- Eats using a spoon and/or needs food to be cut up into small pieces   E: ☐

- Only uses fingers to eat food   S: ☐

- Relies on others to be fed   R: ☐

4. Contact with others

- Initiates social contact and responds to the needs of others   P: ☑

- Aware of others and will seek interaction, but may be more concerned with own needs   E: ☐

- Aware of others but waits for others to make the first social contact   S: ☐

- May not show an awareness of the presence of others unless in direct physical contact   R: ☐

5. Groupwork skills

- Engages with others in a group activity, can take turns with the activity/tools   P: ☑

- Occasionally engages with others in a group, moving in and out of the group at whim   E: ☐

- Aware of others in the group and will work alongside others although tends to focus on own activity   S: ☐

- Does not show awareness of others in the group unless close one-to-one attention is experienced   R: ☐

6. Communication skills

- Is aware of appropriate interaction, can chat coherently and is able to use complex language skills   P: ☑

- Body language may be inappropriate and may not always be coherent, but can use simple language skills   E: ☐

- Responses to verbal interaction may be mainly through body language; comprehension is limited   S: ☐

- Can only respond to direct physical contact from others through touch, eye contact or facial expression   R: ☐

7. Practical activities (craft, domestic chores, gardening)

- Can plan to carry out an activity, hold the goal in mind and work through a familiar sequence; may need help solving problems   P: ☑

- More interested in the making or doing than in the end result, needs prompting to remember purpose, can get distracted   E: ☐

- Activities need to be broken down and presented one step at a time, multisensory stimulation can help to hold the attention   S: ☐

- Unable to 'do' activities, but responds to the close contact of others and experiencing physical sensations   R: ☐

8. Use of objects

- Plans to use and looks for objects that are not visible; may struggle if objects are not in usual/familiar places (i.e. toiletries in a cupboard below washbasin)   P: ☐

- Selects objects appropriately only if in view (i.e. toiletries on a shelf next to washbasin)   E: ☑

- Randomly uses objects as chances upon them; may use Inappropriately   S: ☐

- May grip objects when placed in the hand but will not attempt to use them   R: ☐

9. Looking at a newspaper/magazine

- Comprehends and shows interest in the content, turns the pages and looks at headlines and pictures   P: ☑

- Turns the pages randomly, only attending to items pointed out by others   E: ☐

- Will hold and may feel the paper, but will not turn the pages unless directed and will not show interest in the content   S: ☐

- May grip the paper if it is placed in the hand but may not be able to release grip; or may not take hold of the paper   R: ☐

Select the appropriate PAL Profile to act as a general guide to engaging with the person in a variety of activities.

Complete a PAL Individual Action Plan to act as a specific guide to facilitating personal activities.

	Planned	Exploratory	Sensory	Reflex
TOTAL	9	0	0	0

Case Study 2

Elsie is a retired business woman who owned her own dress shop. Her family have old photographs showing that Elsie was a very well-groomed woman, but sadly she now struggles to dress herself. Elsie is determined to dress herself, but she often looks dishevelled, with petticoats hanging under the hemline of her dress, or put on top of her dress and her hair untidy. Elsie shows that she is aware of her appearance and is often seen tugging at her dress to pull it over the petticoat and smoothing down her hair with her hands.

Elsie has vascular disease and she lives with her daughter and family. They are asking for advice about how they can help Elsie to look smart again without taking away her independence and doing everything for her. Her daughter explains that Elsie relies on her to give her a wash, although she can wipe her face when the soaped cloth is passed to her. She is able to eat her meals using a spoon but struggles to use a knife and fork.

Elsie's family are also concerned that she tries to help with chores but gives up when she cannot find things, and that she tends to blame others, saying someone has not put them away in the right place. For example, Elsie recently became very cross with her granddaughter and accused her of taking her make-up bag, which had actually been tidied away into the top drawer of Elsie's dressing table.

Also, if something else attracts Elsie's attention, she will leave activities unfinished. This causes a great deal of untidiness in the home. Elsie was a very sociable lady but has recently become more withdrawn, although she does respond very positively when people draw her out. She enjoys chatting to her grandchildren when the conversation is about simple and familiar events, although she tends to switch off if more complex topics are discussed. Elsie's granddaughter, Susan, likes to sit and look at *Woman and Home* magazine with her, although Elsie tends only to look at articles when Susan points them out.

Elsie enjoys the social and craft activities at the local day centre which she attends once a week, but does not always stay in the groups, preferring to take a walk every so often and return to the group now and again.

When the Pool Activity Level (PAL) Checklist is completed for Elsie it reveals that, in general, she is able to carry out activities at an exploratory level. It is now possible to use this information in the Activity Profile to help Elsie to use her remaining abilities and to compensate for her disabilities. Elsie has different levels of abilities for some activities. It is therefore also possible to create an Individual Action Plan that recognises these differences.

Pool Activity Level (PAL) Checklist

Name:

Elsie Jones

Date:

1 September 2007

Outcome:

Exploratory

Completing the Checklist: for each activity the statements refer to a different level of ability. Thinking of the last two weeks, tick the statement that represents the person's ability in each activity. There should be only one tick for each activity. If in doubt about which statement to tick, choose the level of ability that represents their average performance over the last two weeks. Make sure you tick one statement for each of the activities.

1. Bathing/Washing

- Can bathe/wash independently, sometimes with a little help to start   P: ☐

- Needs soap put on flannel and one-step-at-a-time directions to wash   E: ☐

- Mainly relies on others but will wipe own face and hands if encouraged   S: ☑

- Totally dependent and needs full assistance to wash or bathe   R: ☐

2. Getting dressed

- Plans what to wear, selects own clothing from cupboards; dresses in correct order   P: ☐

- Needs help to plan what to wear but recognises items and how to wear them; needs help with order of dressing   E: ☑

- Needs help to plan and with order of dressing, but can carry out small activities if someone directs each step S: ☐

- Totally dependent on someone to plan, sequence and complete dressing; may move limbs to assist   R: ☐

3. Eating

- Eats independently and appropriately using the correct cutlery　　　P: ☐

- Eats using a spoon and/or needs food to be cut up into small pieces　　　E: ☑

- Only uses fingers to eat food　　　S: ☐

- Relies on others to be fed　　　R: ☐

4. Contact with others

- Initiates social contact and responds to the needs of others　　　P: ☐

- Aware of others and will seek interaction, but may be more concerned with own needs　　　E: ☐

- Aware of others but waits for others to make the first social contact　　　S: ☑

- May not show an awareness of the presence of others unless in direct physical contact　　　R: ☐

5. Groupwork skills

- Engages with others in a group activity, can take turns with the activity/tools　　　P: ☐

- Occasionally engages with others in a group, moving in and out of the group at whim　　　E: ☑

- Aware of others in the group and will work alongside others although tends to focus on own activity　　　S: ☐

- Does not show awareness of others in the group unless close one-to-one attention is experienced　　　R: ☐

6. Communication skills

- Is aware of appropriate interaction, can chat coherently and is able to use complex language skills   P: ☑

- Body language may be inappropriate and may not always be coherent, but can use simple language skills   E: ☐

- Responses to verbal interaction may be mainly through body language; comprehension is limited   S: ☐

- Can only respond to direct physical contact from others through touch, eye contact or facial expression   R: ☐

7.   Practical activities (craft, domestic chores, gardening)

- Can plan to carry out an activity, hold the goal in mind and work through a familiar sequence; may need help solving problems   P: ☑

- More interested in the making or doing than in the end result, needs prompting to remember purpose, can get distracted   E: ☐

- Activities need to be broken down and presented one step at a time, multisensory stimulation can help to hold the attention   S: ☐

- Unable to 'do' activities, but responds to the close contact of others and experiencing physical sensations   R: ☐

8. Use of objects

- Plans to use and looks for objects that are not visible; may struggle if objects are not in usual/familiar places (i.e. toiletries in a cupboard below washbasin)   P: ☐

- Selects objects appropriately only if in view (i.e. toiletries on a shelf next to washbasin)   E: ☑

- Randomly uses objects as chances upon them; may use inappropriately   S: ☐

- May grip objects when placed in the hand but will not attempt to use them   R: ☐

9. Looking at a newspaper/magazine

- Comprehends and shows interest in the content, turns the pages and looks at headlines and pictures   P: ☐

- Turns the pages randomly, only attending to items pointed out by others   E: ☑

- Will hold and may feel the paper, but will not turn the pages unless directed and will not show interest in the content   S: ☐

- May grip the paper if it is placed in the hand but may not be able to release grip; or may not take hold of the paper   R: ☐

Select the appropriate PAL Profile to act as a general guide to engaging with the person in a variety of activities.

Complete a PAL Individual Action Plan to act as a specific guide to facilitating personal activities.

	Planned	Exploratory	Sensory	Reflex
TOTAL	2	5	2	0

Case Study 3

George is a 45-year-old man with learning disability and early onset Alzheimer's disease. He lives in a small-group-living home but he is beginning to rely increasingly on the support workers for all of his personal care needs. George is only able to carry out activities if the support worker guides him through the steps involved. When George is getting dressed, he needs to be offered clothing items, one at a time, although he is then able to put on some items if someone talks him through the activity. When George has a bath, he relies on the support worker to do everything, only wiping his face and hands with the cloth with the support worker's encouragement.

George used to be a very caring and outgoing person, but now, although he watches the other residents, he does not make the first move to interact with them. When George's friends seek him out, he responds readily, although his understanding of their conversation seems limited and his response is mainly with a big smile and head nodding rather than with words. George's greatest enjoyment seems to be his mealtimes and, when seated with his friends, he will laugh when he hears them laughing. However, most of his attention is focused on his meal, which he eats, using his hands, with great relish.

George used to spend his evenings playing pool with his friends, but this has become difficult because he does not follow the rules of the game and will walk off with the cue. This causes arguments with his friends and George began to spend more time alone, pacing the rooms and picking up items belonging to other residents. When the support workers noticed this, they began to spend more time strolling with him and encouraging him to pick up items that were not contentious. The support workers have noticed that George likes to feel the objects he picks up and that he is drawn to ones with soft textures. They have begun to spend individual time with George, but although they offer to look at the newspaper with him, he seems more interested in the feel of the paper than the content. George does show that he enjoys sitting, holding hands, while they listen together to his favourite music.

Pool Activity Level (PAL) Checklist

Name: Date: Outcome:

George Owen   **1 September 2007**   **Sensory**

Completing the Checklist: for each activity the statements refer to a different level of ability. Thinking of the last two weeks, tick the statement that represents the person's ability in each activity. There should be only one tick for each activity. If in doubt about which statement to tick, choose the level of ability that represents their average performance over the last two weeks. Make sure you tick one statement for each of the activities.

1. Bathing/Washing

- Can bathe/wash independently, sometimes with a little help to start   P: ☐

- Needs soap put on flannel and one-step-at-a-time directions to wash   E: ☐

- Mainly relies on others but will wipe own face and hands if encouraged   S: ☑

- Totally dependent and needs full assistance to wash or bathe   R: ☐

2. Getting dressed

- Plans what to wear, selects own clothing from cupboards; dresses in correct order   P: ☐

- Needs help to plan what to wear but recognises items and how to wear them; needs help with order of dressing   E: ☐

- Needs help to plan and with order of dressing, but can carry out small activities if someone directs each step   S: ☑

- Totally dependent on someone to plan, sequence and complete dressing; may move limbs to assist   R: ☐

3. Eating

- Eats independently and appropriately using the correct cutlery   P: ☐

- Eats using a spoon and/or needs food to be cut up into small pieces   E: ☐

- Only uses fingers to eat food   S: ☑

- Relies on others to be fed   R: ☐

4. Contact with others

- Initiates social contact and responds to the needs of others   P: ☐

- Aware of others and will seek interaction, but may be more concerned with own needs   E: ☐

- Aware of others but waits for others to make the first social contact   S: ☑

- May not show an awareness of the presence of others unless in direct physical contact   R: ☐

5. Groupwork skills

- Engages with others in a group activity, can take turns with the activity/tools   P: ☐

- Occasionally engages with others in a group, moving in and out of the group at whim   E: ☐

- Aware of others in the group and will work alongside others although tends to focus on own activity S: ☑

- Does not show awareness of others in the group unless close one-to-one attention is experienced   R: ☐

6. Communication skills

- Is aware of appropriate interaction, can chat coherently and is able to use complex language skills   P: ☐

- Body language may be inappropriate and may not always be coherent, but can use simple language skills   E: ☐

- Responses to verbal interaction may be mainly through body language; comprehension is limited   S: ☑

- Can only respond to direct physical contact from others through touch, eye contact or facial expression   R: ☐

7. Practical activities (craft, domestic chores, gardening)

- Can plan to carry out an activity, hold the goal in mind and work through a familiar sequence; may need help solving problems   P: ☐

- More interested in the making or doing than in the end result, needs prompting to remember purpose, can get distracted   E: ☐

- Activities need to be broken down and presented one step at a time, multisensory stimulation can help to hold the attention   S: ☑

- Unable to 'do' activities, but responds to the close contact of others and experiencing physical sensations   R: ☐

8. Use of objects

- Plans to use and looks for objects that are not visible; may struggle if objects are not in usual/familiar places (i.e. toiletries in a cupboard below washbasin)   P: ☐

- Selects objects appropriately only if in view (i.e. toiletries on a shelf next to washbasin)   E: ☐

- Randomly uses objects as chances upon them; may use inappropriately   S: ☑

- May grip objects when placed in the hand but will not attempt to use them   R: ☐

9. Looking at a newspaper/magazine

- Comprehends and shows interest in the content, turns the pages and looks at headlines and pictures   P: ☐

- Turns the pages randomly, only attending to items pointed out by others   E: ☐

- Will hold and may feel the paper, but will not turn the pages unless directed and will not show interest in the content   S: ☑

- May grip the paper if it is placed in the hand but may not be able to release grip; or may not take hold of the paper   R: ☐

Select the appropriate PAL Profile to act as a general guide to engaging with the person in a variety of activities.

Complete a PAL Individual Action Plan to act as a specific guide to facilitating personal activities.

	Planned	Exploratory	Sensory	Reflex
TOTAL	0	0	9	0

Case Study 4

Gertie lives on a long-stay hospital ward. She has severe dementia caused by a combination of Alzheimer's disease and vascular disease that has resulted in her experiencing a series of strokes. Gertie relies on the nursing staff for all of her care needs. Gertie does not seem to understand anything that is said to her and most of her contact with others is with people who come up close to her, when she will screw up the muscles of her face and gaze into their eyes. The nursing staff enable her to sit in the group singing activities, and she does become more animated when the music is playing, although she does not seem to be aware of the other group members unless those nearest to her are holding her hands. Gertie will also grasp firmly anything that is placed into the palm of her hands and sometimes she has trouble letting go again.

Gertie loves to see children and animals, and will make crooning noises when they visit the ward. She dislikes sudden loud noises and will shout angrily if they disturb her. Gertie used to work in a flower shop and she still loves to look at, and smell, flowers when they are brought to her.

The nursing staff want to help Gertie to engage with her surroundings as much as she can.

Pool Activity Level (PAL) Checklist

Name:
Gertie Lawson

Date:
1 September 2007

Outcome:
Reflex

Completing the Checklist: for each activity the statements refer to a different level of ability. Thinking of the last two weeks, tick the statement that represents the person's ability in each activity. There should be only one tick for each activity. If in doubt about that statement to tick, choose the level of ability that represents their average performance over the last two weeks. Make sure you tick one statement for each of the activities.

1. Bathing/Washing

- Can bathe/wash independently, sometimes with a little help to start   P: ☐

- Needs soap put on flannel and one-step-at-a-time directions to wash   E: ☐

- Mainly relies on others but will wipe own face and hands if encouraged   S: ☐

- Totally dependent and needs full assistance to wash or bathe   R: ☑

2. Getting dressed

- Plans what to wear, selects own clothing from cupboards; dresses in correct order   P: ☐

- Needs help to plan what to wear but recognises items and how to wear them; needs help with order of dressing   E: ☐

- Needs help to plan and with order of dressing, but can carry out small activities if someone directs each step   S: ☐

- Totally dependent on someone to plan, sequence and complete dressing; may move limbs to assist   R: ☑

3. Eating

- Eats independently and appropriately using the correct cutlery   P: ☐

- Eats using a spoon and/or needs food to be cut up into small pieces   E: ☐

- Only uses fingers to eat food   S: ☐

- Relies on others to be fed   R: ☑

4. Contact with others

- Initiates social contact and responds to the needs of others   P: ☐

- Aware of others and will seek interaction, but may be more concerned with own needs   E: ☐

- Aware of others but waits for others to make the first social contact   S: ☐

- May not show an awareness of the presence of others unless in direct physical contact   R: ☑

5. Groupwork skills

- Engages with others in a group activity, can take turns with the activity/tools   P: ☐

- Occasionally engages with others in a group, moving in and out of the group at whim   E: ☐

- Aware of others in the group and will work alongside others although tends to focus on own activity   S: ☐

- Does not show awareness of others in the group unless close one-to-one attention is experienced   R: ☑

6. Communication skills

- Is aware of appropriate interaction, can chat coherently and is able to use complex language skills   P: ☐

- Body language may be inappropriate and may not always be coherent, but can use simple language skills   E: ☐

- Responses to verbal interaction may be mainly through body language; comprehension is limited   S: ☐

- Can only respond to direct physical contact from others through touch, eye contact or facial expression   R: ☑

7. Practical activities (craft, domestic chores, gardening)

- Can plan to carry out an activity, hold the goal in mind and work through a familiar sequence; may need help solving problems   P: ☐

- More interested in the making or doing than in the end result, needs prompting to remember purpose, can get distracted   E: ☐

- Activities need to be broken down and presented one step at a time, multisensory stimulation can help to hold the attention   S: ☐

- Unable to 'do' activities, but responds to the close contact of others and experiencing physical sensations   R: ☑

8. Use of objects

- Plans to use and looks for objects that are not visible; may struggle if objects are not in usual/familiar places (i.e. toiletries in a cupboard below washbasin)   P: ☐

- Selects objects appropriately only if in view (i.e. toiletries on a shelf next to washbasin)   E: ☐

- Randomly uses objects as chances upon them; may use inappropriately   S: ☐

- May grip objects when placed in the hand but will not attempt to use them   R: ☑

9. Looking at a newspaper/magazine

- Comprehends and shows interest in the content, turns
  the pages and looks at headlines and pictures   P: ☐

- Turns the pages randomly, only attending to items
  pointed out by others   E: ☐

- Will hold and may feel the paper, but will not turn
  the pages unless directed and will not show interest in
  the content   S: ☐

- May grip the paper if it is placed in the hand but may not
  be able to release grip; or may not take hold of the paper   R: ☑

Select the appropriate PAL Profile to act as a general guide to engaging with the person in a variety of activities.

Complete a PAL Individual Action Plan to act as a specific guide to facilitating personal activities.

	Planned	Exploratory	Sensory	Reflex
TOTAL	0	0	0	9

These case studies give examples of how the behaviour of the person can be recorded using the PAL Checklist to identify their level of ability. The user of the PAL Instrument is then prompted to select the appropriate PAL Profile to act as a general guide to engaging with the person in a variety of activities. Including the information gained from the person's Life History Profile enhances this information

In addition to the general PAL Profile, the user is also able to complete a PAL Individual Action Plan, which acts as a specific guide to facilitating personal activities. In three of the case studies, the level of ability in each of the activities on the Checklist is the same throughout. Therefore completion of the Individual Action Plan would use the same level of ability information for all three personal care activities. In Case Study 2, however, the person is functioning at different levels of ability in different activity. The Individual Action Plan would reflect this by having a record of how to engage the person in the activity at the relevant level of ability as revealed by the Checklist. An example of how to complete the Individual Action Plan in these circumstances is given in Chapter 6.

Chapter 6

Planning Interventions

Completing the Pool Activity Level (PAL) Profile

When a care giver helps a person with cognitive impairment to carry out an activity it is important that the care giver does not do too much because this will undermine the person's self-confidence and could result in the person becoming more dependent. Equally, it is important that care givers do not do too little because the well-being of the person will be undermined if he or she struggles to carry out the activities. It is therefore useful to plan the best way of helping the person with cognitive impairments to carry out activities. Staff in residential homes will be familiar with care plans, although these sometimes focus on the activities to be done rather than on the method of helping the person to carry them out. Although planning care-giving in a person's own home where a family member, for example, is the carer might seem excessive, it is essential in clarifying the most effective way of enabling the person being cared for. Planning in this way also promotes a consistent approach from all care givers, whether they are staff, relatives or friends.

The Pool Activity Level (PAL) Profile assists care givers to translate an understanding of the level of ability of the person with cognitive impairment into practical methods of helping him or her to engage in activities. There are four PAL Profiles, one for each activity level. The care giver should select the Profile that is revealed as appropriate following completion of the PAL Checklist. Each Profile describes how to assist the person by positioning objects that are needed to carry out the activity and by giving verbal or physical directions. The objectives and characteristics of activities that are likely to be meaningful to a person at the level of ability are also described in each Profile.

In addition, some information about the person's likely abilities and limitations is given. This can be helpful in aiding the care giver to build on the person's strengths and to compensate for his or her limitations. In the Checklist examples, John is at a 'planned' level of ability. As the PAL Profile reveals, this means that he can explore different ways of carrying out an activity and can carry out activities as long as the objects he needs are in their usual place and the end result of the activity is obvious, so that he knows what he is working towards and when he has finished. However, John may not be able to solve any problems that arise and, for example, may not be able to look for any objects that he needs to carry out the activity if they are not where he expects to find them.

The Profile for Elsie reveals that she can carry out very familiar activities in very familiar environments but may have a problem with those that involve a complex series of stages, such as getting dressed. So although she is completing the activity of getting dressed, and wishes to do this alone, she is not able to carry out the steps involved in the correct sequence and therefore the end result is haphazard. Elsie also tends to start activities but not finish them and this may be because she has difficulty fixing an end result in her mind at the beginning.

The Checklist example for George reveals that he is able to carry out activities at a 'sensory' level of ability. The Profile indicates that, at this level of ability, George is likely to be responding to bodily sensations rather than engaging in the 'doing' of activities. Any activities he is helped to carry out successfully will be those that are simple one-step ones, or those that have been broken down into single stages. At this level, George is likely to be limited in his ability to initiate social contact and will be reliant on others making the first move.

Gertie only engages with her surroundings when there is a direct impact on her own senses. She does not actively seek engagement and so is very reliant on others to ensure that she receives opportunities for stimulation and fulfilment. The Profile for Gertie's 'reflex' level of ability shows that she can respond in a reflex way to direct sensory stimulation and through this she can become more aware of herself and her surroundings. At this level, Gertie may have difficulty attending to, or may become agitated by, complex and multi sensory messages.

Completion of the appropriate PAL Profile will guide care givers in presenting all activities that the person may wish to undertake in a way that maximises the opportunity for meaningful engagement. The example Checklists are developed here so that the Profiles may be clarified.

Blank copies of the PAL Instrument, including the Checklist, Profile, Individual Action Plan and the Outcome Sheet, can be found at the back of Part 1 of this book. They may be photocopied for your use with the people for whom you care.

Pool Activity Level (PAL) Profile

Name: John Porter   **Date: 1 September 2007**

Planned Activity Level

Likely abilities

Can explore different ways of carrying out an activity

Can work towards completing an activity with a tangible result

Can look in obvious places for any equipment

Likely limitations

May not be able to solve problems that arise

May not be able to understand complex sentences

May not search beyond the usual places for equipment

Method of engagement

Activity objectives	To enable *John* to take control of the activity and to master the steps involved
Position of objects	Ensure that equipment and materials are in their usual, familiar places
Verbal directions	Explain activity using short sentences, avoiding using connecting phrases such as 'and', 'but', 'therefore', or 'if'
Demonstrated directions	Show *John* how to avoid possible errors
Working with others	*John* is able to make the first contact and should be encouraged to initiate social contact
Activity characteristics	There is a goal or end product, with a set process, or 'recipe', to achieve it. An element of competition with others is motivating

The Profile shows that John will remain independent for as long as possible, given the nature of his condition, if his surroundings remain constant so that the familiar positioning of items will act as cues for the next stage in activities. John will also be able to carry out less familiar activities so long as he is made aware of the aim of an activity and the method is made clear. This clarity will help John to feel confident and secure when he is carrying out activities so that his self-esteem will not be undermined.

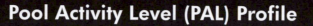

Pool Activity Level (PAL) Profile

Name: Elsie Jones   **Date: 1 September 2007**

EXPLORATORY ACTIVITY LEVEL

Likely abilities

Can carry out very familiar activities in familiar surroundings

Enjoys the experience of doing an activity more than the end result

Can carry out more complex activities if they are broken down into two-to-three step stages

Likely limitations

May not have an end result in mind when starts an activity

May not recognise when the activity is completed

Relies on cues such as diaries, newspaper, lists and labels

Method of engagement

Activity objectives	To enable *Elsie* to experience the sensation of doing the activity rather than focusing on the end result
Position of objects	Ensure that equipment and materials are in the line of vision
Verbal directions	Explain activity using short simple sentences. Avoid using connecting phrases such as 'and', 'but', 'therefore', or 'if'
Demonstrated directions	Break the activity into two to three steps at a time
Working with others	Others must approach *Elsie* and make the first contact
Activity characteristics	There is no pressure to perform to a set of rules, or to achieve an end result. There is an element of creativity and spontaneity

The Profile shows that the care giver needs to guide Elsie to carry out any activities in stages. Elsie wishes to retain her independence in getting dressed and at the same time to return to her previous standard of grooming. The care giver can facilitate this by helping her sort out her wardrobe and drawers so that items are kept together and are labelled. This may help Elsie to select garments appropriately. In addition, Elsie may enjoy the care giver assisting her while she dresses if the focus is on choosing what to wear and looking at the colours, patterns and texture of the clothes. This is likely to have more meaning for Elsie than the actual act of dressing. It will be important that the care giver helps Elsie to make the finishing touches of hair combing, make-up and jewellery. Elsie can be reassured about her appearance by being encouraged to check herself in a mirror.

This information will help Elsie's family to enable Elsie to experience feelings of self-confidence and self-esteem, because she will be aware that her appearance meets her own standards, while at the same time her independence has not been taken away: she has been enabled to carry out the dressing activity at her own level of ability.

Pool Activity Level (PAL) Profile

Name: George Owen   **Date: 1 September 2007**

Sensory Activity Level

Likely abilities

Is likely to be responding to bodily sensations

Can be guided to carry out single-step activities

Can carry out more complex activities if they are broken down into one step at a time

Likely limitations

May not have any conscious plan to carry out a movement to achieve a particular end result

May be relying on others to make social contact

Method of engagement

Activity objectives	To enable *George* to experience the effect of the activity on the senses
Position of objects	Ensure that *George* becomes aware of equipment and materials by making bodily contact
Verbal directions	Limit requests to carry out actions to the naming of actions and objects e.g. 'Lift your arm', 'Hold the brush'
Demonstrated directions	Show *George* the action on the object. Break the activity down into one step at a time
Working with others	Others must approach *George* and make the first contact. Use touch and *George*'s name to sustain the social contact
Activity characteristics	The activity is used as an opportunity for a sensory experience. This may be multi-sensory and repetitive

As we see in George's case study (Chapter 5) George is engaging with his surroundings by enjoying the sensations, particularly of touch. The care givers have recognised the importance of this to George and are providing him with opportunities for interacting with them through the medium of touch.

This Profile will help care givers to realise that it is important for George to enjoy being involved in the process of carrying out the activity, rather than in the end result. It will also help them to recognise that, despite his disability, George still has many abilities and that he can do activities which do not involve more than one step. There are many such activities, including sweeping, polishing and wiping surfaces.

When activities are presented to George in this way, he is likely to regain his sense of being a part of things in his home and, by his actions, of being able to make things happen.

Pool Activity Level (PAL) Profile

Name: Gertie Lawson   **Date: 1 September 2007**

Reflex Activity Level

Likely abilities

Can make reflex responses to direct sensory stimulation

Can increase awareness of self, and others, by engagement of senses

May respond to social engagement through the use of body language

Likely limitations

May be in a subliminal or subconscious state

May have difficulty organising the multiple sensations that are being experienced

May become agitated in an environment that is over-stimulating

Method of engagement

Activity objectives	To arouse *Gertie* to a conscious awareness of self
Position of objects	Stimulate area of body being targeted, e.g. stroke *Gertie*'s arm before placing it in a sleeve
Verbal directions	Limit spoken directions to movement directions, i.e., 'Lift', 'Hold', 'Open'
Demonstrated directions	Guide movements by touching the relevant body part
Working with others	Maintain eye contact, make maximum use of facial expression, gestures and body posture for a nonverbal conversation. Use social actions which can be imitated, e.g. smiling, waving, shaking hands
Activity characteristics	The activity is in response to direct selective sensory stimulation

Gertie's Profile reveals how important it is that others approach her and make contact with her by stimulating her sense of hearing, sight, smell, taste or touch. When this happens, Gertie obviously responds, so planning to make it happen frequently will give Gertie an increased opportunity for engaging with others and her surroundings.

These are examples of how a Pool Activity Level (PAL) Profile can be used to address one aspect of a person's life. Most care givers, though, are concerned with much more than just one activity. They want to know how to help the person they care for to undertake a range of activities and thus to maintain a stimulating and fulfilling life.

The Profile describes *how*, in general, to help a person with cognitive impairment according to different levels of ability. The final stage of using the PAL Profile is to work out *what* activities should be provided or encouraged. This information would then be entered in the final box on the Profile form. Chapter 9 describes how to use the information from the Life History Profile to ensure that activities that are meaningful to the person are entered on this form.

Care givers often seek specific guidance for enabling the person they care for to realise his or her potential for carrying out personal care activities, such as bathing, dining or dressing. The Pool Activity Level (PAL) Individual Action Plan has been designed to be used in this way so that a person with cognitive impairment is facilitated to carry out a range of personal care activities using his or her abilities.

COMPLETING THE POOL ACTIVITY LEVEL (PAL) INDIVIDUAL ACTION PLAN

A person with cognitive impairment will have some cognitive skills that are still intact. This will vary depending on the area of damage in the brain. In any case the ability to carry out activities does not always rely on the integrity of the brain; familiarity with the activity and the activity environment, and the type of support the person receives while carrying out the activities, will either facilitate or undermine the person's ability. It is often apparent that a person does have different levels of ability in different activities. Completion of the PAL Checklist can be helpful in revealing this. The care giver is guided to note the level of ability of the person in the activities of dressing, bathing and dining and then refer to the Individual Action Plan Guidance Notes. These reveal a method for facilitating the person's engagement in each of the three activities.

Transferring the information from the Guidance Notes onto the Individual Action Plan can be completed in several ways. The user can photocopy the Guidance Notes and then cut them out and stick them onto the Individual Action Plan, or the user may prefer to handwrite the information. If there is access to a computer, the user may transfer the PAL Instrument onto it and use the cut and paste facility to enter the relevant information onto the Individual Action Plan.

Because social and psychological factors also play an important role in determining an individual's ability to carry out an activity, the user is also encouraged to consider these when completing the Individual Action Plan. By referring to the person's Life History Profile, and by observing the person's responses when assisting him or her to carry out an activity, it is possible also to pay attention to the person's preferences and to plan to accommodate these.

In the Pool Activity Level (PAL) Checklist examples (Chapter 5) it was revealed that Elsie, in general, is able to carry out activities at an exploratory level. This information was used to complete the Activity Profile to help Elsie to use her remaining abilities and to compensate for her disabilities. It was also noted, though, that Elsie has differing levels of abilities for different activities. It is therefore also possible to create an Individual Action Plan that recognises these differences.

Pool Activity Level (PAL) Individual Action Plan

Name: Elsie Jones   **Date: 1 September 2007**

Dressing

Favourite garments Dresses, cardigans
Preferred routine Dress after breakfast, in bedroom
Grooming likes and dislikes Does not like hair to be left loose or to wear slides. Wears lipstick and blusher (in top drawer of dressing table)
Method: Exploratory Activity Level

- Encourage discussion about the clothing to be worn for the day: is it suitable for the weather or the occasion, is it a favourite item?

- Spend time colour-matching items of clothing and select accessories

- Break down the activity into manageable chunks: help lay the clothes out in order, for example, so that underclothing is at the top of the pile

- Encourage Elsie to check her appearance in the mirror

Bathing

Favourite toiletries Lavender bath foam, Palmolive soap, lavender talcum powder
Preferred routine Bath at 9.30 p.m., then wears nightgown and dressing gown and has hot chocolate while watching 10 p.m. news before going to bed
Bathing likes and dislikes Likes bath to be full but not too hot. Prefers to use a sponge for her body and a cloth for her face
Method: Sensory Activity Level

- Prepare the bathroom and run the bath water for Elsie

- Make the bathroom warm and inviting – play music, use scented oils or bubble bath, have candles lit and placed safely out of reach

- Break down the activity into one step at a time and give Elsie simple directions: 'Rub the soap on the cloth, rub your arm, rinse your arm, rub your chest, rinse your chest…'

Dining

Favourite foods Casseroles, soup, treacle pudding

Preferred routine Main meal at lunch time, tea at 5 p.m. and a light supper at 8.30 p.m. before bathing

Dining likes and dislikes Does not like spicy foods. Prefers small portions and likes food to be cut up

Method: Exploratory Activity Level

- Store cutlery and crockery in view and encourage Elsie to select own tools for dining

- Offer food using simple choices

- Create a social atmosphere using, for example, table decorations and music, and promote conversation

Chapter 7

Implementing Interventions

ACTIVITIES

When considering the range of activities in which we all engage, it may be helpful to split them into three main categories: personal care activities; domestic activities; such as cleaning, cooking and gardening; and leisure interests. A person with cognitive impairment can be helped to carry out any of these activities using the PAL Profile, and the Individual Action Plan pays particular attention to the personal care activities

Most care givers find that there is insufficient time for the person they care for to carry out all activities at his or her own level of ability, particularly when the pace of the person is slowed. For many family care givers, the demands of enabling the person they care for to work through an activity can be physically and emotionally exhausting. Attempting to work to one's full potential in all areas of daily life will be equally exhausting to the person with cognitive impairment. For care givers in communal settings, such as residential homes or hospitals, there are often not enough staff to allow this amount of individual time with people.

The solution is to give priority to the activities that have the most importance for the person with cognitive impairment, so that he or she is able to do as much as is possible in those aspects, while helping him or her to conserve energy by giving increased assistance in areas that are felt to be of lesser importance. For example, Elsie, who has always paid a lot of attention to her physical appearance, may be enabled to carry out grooming activities to her full potential, but domestic chores such as making the bed can be done for her. George, who shows great enthusiasm for the social and the dining aspects of mealtimes and has begun to respond to the sensory experiences around him, may prefer to accept assistance with his bathing and dressing needs, so that he has more time and energy to enjoy engaging with others through these sensory opportunities.

Care givers who are close relatives or friends will have a wealth of information about the life history and the personality of the person with cognitive impairment. The PAL Life History Profile (Chapter 4) is a useful guide to gathering and recording this type of information and is a valuable starting point in planning which occupations will be of most interest. If the person is living in a communal setting, the care giver can share this information with the staff so that the most appropriate occupations are offered. If the person lives at home with a care giver, and services such as home care are provided, this information can be also shared with those service providers.

Care givers sometimes feel that it is inappropriate to encourage the person with cognitive impairment to carry out an occupation that cannot be performed at as high a standard as was previously. However, if the person is still interested in the activity, it is likely that he or she will still enjoy the opportunity to carry it out and, if the person is concerned about the standard of the final outcome, by presenting the activity using the guidelines in the PAL Profile the person will be able to engage with the activity in manageable stages. For many people with cognitive impairment, it is not the final end product that is as important as the opportunity to engage in the process of doing the activity. When care givers recognise this they can place less emphasis on what has been achieved in terms of final product than on what has been achieved in terms of experiencing the activity.

The knowledge of a person's interests and familiar routines, together with an understanding of how he or she best carries out activities, can be utilised to ensure occupations are engaged in that are unique to the individual. As the person is provided with opportunities to become meaningfully occupied, it may well be that his or her cognitive and functional ability will improve. Adopting a facilitating approach should help the person's level of ability to be sustained for longer. Even, when a person's ability level decreases, as is possible given the nature of some of the conditions causing cognitive impairment, it is unlikely that the person's interests will change. Therefore these may continue, using the Action Plan for the new level. For example, John may be helped to engage in gardening activities using the PAL Action Plan at a planned level of ability. In the future, he may lose some of these abilities and it may become appropriate still to present gardening opportunities to him, but to use the PAL Action Plan for an exploratory level of ability that will give guidance on how to continue to facilitate his gardening interest.

It is proposed that it is possible to take any activity that a person is interested in and use the appropriate Action Plan to present it at the right level for that individual. Examples of some typical activities, which can be presented at either a planned, exploratory, sensory or reflex level, are presented on the next pages. These are intended to give a flavour of how the information in the Action Plan can be translated into everyday practice.

Activity: Gardening

Planned Activity Level

- Plan a planting activity by looking through seed catalogues and gardening magazines, or visiting a gardening centre.

- Encourage the person to take charge of getting the equipment off the gardening shelf/trolley and planting the plants out in the garden or tub.

- Hand over the responsibility for watering or weeding (the person may need reminding).

- Encourage the person to clean up after the activity is completed and to put away tools in the appropriate places.

Exploratory Activity Level

- Encourage the person to be creative with the planting arrangement, select unusual containers and spend time discussing which plants will look attractive in them.

- Arrange a workspace close to where the equipment is on view. Ensure that items are obvious: keep plant labels and the potting-compost bag turned toward the person so that the writing and pictures are visible.

- Break down the activity into manageable chunks: suggest to the person that he or she uses a trowel or old spoon to fill the tray or bowl with potting compost; when that is accomplished suggest that the plants be placed in the container and, when that is achieved, suggest that the person fills a watering can and waters the plants.

- Create a social occasion; perhaps use the activity as an opportunity to reminisce about previous gardens or to discuss favourite plants.

Sensory Activity Level

- Prepare a table with the planting equipment.

- Encourage the person to use his or her hands to put the potting compost into the containers. Spend time crumbling it and smoothing it with the fingers.

- Plant scented herbs. Encourage the person to crush some leaves in his or her fingers and to smell or taste them.

- Enter watering into the person's weekly planner or diary and accompany him or her on this activity.

Reflex Activity Level

- Position the person next to you when you carry out the planting activity. Ensure that he or she is comfortable and can see what you are doing.

- Keep equipment that is not being used out of the person's line of vision.

- Offer a plant to the person to smell by placing your fingers over theirs and, together, gently crush the plant. Raise the person's hand to his or her face and suggest that they 'smell' the plant.

- Use your body language of smiling and nodding to reinforce that this is a pleasant experience for you too.

Activity: Preparing a fruit salad

Planned Activity Level

- Use a recipe card with a picture of the end result.

- Encourage the person to follow the directions on the recipe card to make the fruit juice base for the salad.

- Encourage the person to take charge of cutting the fruit up and arranging it in the bowl.

Exploratory Activity Level

- Use a tin of fruit as a base for the salad so that the juice does not have to be made. Add fresh orange juice to it so that there is sufficient juice. Have a selection of fresh fruit to add to the base.

- Arrange a workplace close to where the equipment is on view. Ensure that items needed are obvious: keep the tin of fruit and the orange juice container turned so that the labels are visible.

- Encourage the person to be creative about selecting the fruit and the container to be used, and spend time discussing which colours of fruit will look attractive.

- Break down the activity into manageable chunks: suggest to the person that he or she opens the tin and empties it into the salad container; when that is accomplished, suggest that you will peel the fruit while the person chops it.

- Create a social occasion out of the activity: use it as an opportunity to reminisce about family meals or to discuss favourite foods.

Sensory Activity Level

- Prepare the table with an orange, apple, pear and seedless grapes, a container and the cutlery. Open a tin of pineapple to act as a base for the salad.

- Encourage the person to handle each piece of fruit, to feel the texture of the skin and to smell it.

- Break down the activity into one step at a time: peel the orange and suggest that the person split the segments while you chop the apple and pear. When this is accomplished, suggest to the person that he or she picks the grapes off the stem and puts them into the container with the rest of the salad.

- When finished, encourage the person to smell and to lick his or her fingers and to enjoy the aroma and the look of the fruit salad.

Reflex Activity Level

- Position the person next to you when you prepare the fruit salad. Ensure that the person is comfortable and can see what you are doing.

- Only have on view the piece of fruit which you are preparing; keep the fruit and equipment that is not in immediate use out of the person's line of vision.

- Place a piece of soft fruit, such as a banana or kiwi fruit, in the person's hand and assist him or her to hold it by placing your fingers over theirs. Raise the person's hand to his or her face and encourage them to smell and taste.

- Use your body language of smiling and nodding to reinforce that this is a pleasant experience for you too.

Chapter 8

Seeing Results

AIMS AND RATIONALE OF THE PAL INSTRUMENT

The purpose of this Guide is not simply to encourage readers to embark on a purely academic exercise to find out the level of a person's cognitive disability and the corresponding level of functional ability. Rather, it is intended to enable care givers to enhance the experience of the person with cognitive impairment through an increased understanding of his or her abilities and the provision of appropriately presented occupations. When this occurs there is often an effect on the person's psychological, social and cognitive experience. In other words, the person may not only have enhanced feelings of self-confidence and self-esteem, he or she may also experience a higher level of thinking and reasoning and of communication with others.

THE PERSON-CENTRED APPROACH

A person-centred approach is possible because of the close relationship between cognition, feeling and action. It is helpful to view these three states as the points of a triangle, each being separate from, but also interrelating with, the others. For example, low feelings cause every person to think, reason and act less efficiently. Equally, negative thoughts cause low feelings and can stifle the ability to act effectively; and a lack of action can lead to low mood and negative thoughts. Knowledge of this triangle can be used by care givers to raise the level of ability in all three areas by focusing on the two that are the most easily influenced in a person with cognitive impairment: feelings and actions.

This concept is at the heart of a person-centred approach to caring for people with dementia (Kitwood 1990), which is grounded in the theory that dementia is a disability caused not only by neurological impairment but also by a damaging social psychology, undermining interactions with others and a lack of opportunity for engagement in meaningful occupation.

Actions and activities can be used by care givers as a vehicle for interaction. Communication which achieves close contact between the care giver and the person with cognitive impairment will enhance the person's mood. In addition, if the activity or action is facilitated at the right level for the individual, feelings of self-confidence and self-esteem will also be experienced as the person is able to participate successfully. This type of success is not unusual and many care givers report that the person they care for seems at times to improve beyond expectation.

RECORDING THE RESULTS OF ACTIVITIES

Giving real-life 'before and after' descriptions is an interesting way for care givers to describe the results of their activity with an individual; but a story in itself may not be sufficient to convince others of the potential for improvement. Hard facts are sometimes needed. That is why it is helpful to keep records that show the progress of the person with cognitive impairment, not only in their actions by recording what they can or cannot do, but also in their experiences by recording what they seem to be feeling as portrayed by their behaviour.

THE PAL OUTCOME SHEET

The PAL Outcome Sheet is one simple method of record-keeping, which uses a numerical score to record the response of a person to the activity in which they have been engaged. It makes statements of behaviours that are likely to be observed when people are engaging in activities at each of the four activity levels. This helps the care giver to identify easily whether the person responded as expected, and whether his or her experience was a positive one. The Checklist can be used to monitor the progress of the person over a period of time, but it can also be used for care givers to monitor their own progress – to determine whether they are getting it right.

Users of the PAL Outcome Sheet have found it helpful to use one sheet for a specific activity and to have three to four sheets for each person that they are caring for. It can be useful to copy the sheet onto different colour paper for each activity, for example: blue for dressing activity, green for gardening activity, and yellow for art and craft activity.

Care givers of people with cognitive impairment in their own home may feel that record keeping is not for them, that it is only necessary for hospitals and homes. But record keeping need not be complex or time-consuming and it can have two major impacts on the experience of the people being cared for. First, if care givers from all settings keep records, then they can contribute to research into effective ways of working with people with cognitive impairments. Second, if care givers keep records and are actively seeking improvements in the experience of the person or people they care for, then they are maintaining an attitude of expectation rather than one of acceptance that there is no scope for improvement. The negative culture of assuming an inevitable decline of the person with cognitive impairment where the cause is viewed as progressive, such as in Alzheimer's disease, is now held to be harmful itself – it may become a self-fulfilling prophecy. If care givers and the person being cared for accept this assumption, the person's psychological well-being is undermined and this can adversely affect the person's physical health and functional ability. An expectation that positive care giving can have a healing effect, where the person may improve to a higher level of cognition and ability, will change the whole culture of caring for this group of people.

REFERENCE

Kitwood, T. (1990) 'The Dialectics of Dementia: With Particular Reference to Alzheimer's Disease.' *Ageing and Society 10*, 177–196.

Chapter 9

The Pool Activity Level (PAL) Instrument

DIRECTIONS

Completing the PAL Life History Profile

The aim of this is to gather and record information that will improve the opportunities for the person with cognitive impairment to engage in meaningful activity. Completion of the Life History Profile will depend on what sections are relevant, what information is available and what the person wishes to be recorded. The headings in each section are intended as a guide. This is likely to be an ongoing process rather than a once-only activity, and can become a meaningful activity for the person in itself.

Completing the PAL Checklist

Consider how the person with cognitive impairment generally functions when carrying out the activities described in the Checklist. If you are unsure, observe the person in the situations over a period of two weeks. If the person lives in a group setting, such as a home, you might need to ask other care givers for their observations too.

For each activity, the statements refer to a different level of ability. Thinking of the last two weeks, tick the statement that represents the person's ability in each activity. There should be only one tick for each activity. If in doubt about which statement to tick, choose the level of ability that represents the person's average performance over the last two weeks. Make sure you tick only one statement for each of the activities.

Interpreting the Checklist

People do not fit neatly into boxes, and the PAL Instrument is designed to describe people in simple terms so that it is widely applicable. Add up the number of ticks for each activity level and enter the number in the total box at the end of the Checklist. You should find that there is a majority of ticks in one of the levels. This indicates which Activity Profile to select. If the number of ticks is evenly divided between two activity levels, assume that the person is currently functioning at the lower level of ability for the purpose of selecting the Activity Profile, but ensure that the person has opportunity to move into the higher level of ability.

Completing the Activity Profile

This is a general description of the environment in which the person is likely to best engage in activities. The box at the end of the Activity Profile should be completed by referring to the information gathered and recorded in the Life History Profile. This is how the general nature of the Activity Profile becomes individualised.

Completing the Individual Action Plan

Note the level of ability of the person in the activities of dressing, bathing and dining that have been revealed on the PAL Checklist and refer to the Individual Action Plan Guidance Notes. These reveal a method for facilitating the person's engagement in each of the three activities. Enter the methods of facilitating the engagement of the person with cognitive disability onto the relevant section of the Individual Action Plan.

Transferring the information from the Guidance Notes onto the Individual Action Plan can be completed in several ways. The user can photocopy the Guidance Notes and then cut and stick them onto the Individual Action Plan, or the user may prefer to handwrite the information. If there is access to a computer, the user may transfer the PAL Instrument onto it and use the cut and paste facility to enter the relevant information onto the Individual Action Plan.

Completing the Outcome Sheet

Use one Outcome Sheet for each activity engaged in. You may find it useful to copy or print these onto different colour paper for different activities, for example: green for dining, blue for a particular leisure activity, or yellow for getting dressed.

Enter the date and the type of activity in the appropriate boxes and score each of the statements with 0, 1 or 2 according to whether the person never, sometimes or always engages in the activity in the way that the statement describes.

You can total the scores as an overall indicator of engagement and also use scores for individual statements to assist you with reviewing the success of the activity and with planning how you will continue.

Pool Activity Level (PAL) Personal History Profile

The purpose of a Personal History Profile is to enable carers to recognise the person as a unique individual and not to see only the person's disability. By finding out about all that the person has experienced it is possible to have a better understanding of the person's behaviour now. It also gives care workers who do not know the person very well topics of conversation that will have meaning for the person.

Putting together the Profile should be an enjoyable project that the person with dementia, relatives and care workers can all join in together, encouraging life review and reminiscence. The information gained from the Personal History Profile informs the PAL Activity Profile by guiding activity selection.

The questions in the Profile are very general, designed to cater for all people regardless of age or sex. Some questions may be irrelevant, so just ignore these!

If you can include any photographs to add to this Profile please write on the reverse:

- the person's name

- who is in the photo

- where and when it was taken.

If you are worried about the photographs getting lost or damaged, you could get them photocopied.

Pool Activity Level (PAL) Personal History Profile

What is your name?   **When were you born?**

Childhood

Where were you born?

What are your family members' names?

What were your family members' occupations?

Where did you live?

Which schools did you attend?

What was your favourite subject?

Did you have any family pets?

What were their names?

Adolescence

When did you leave school?

Where did you work?

What did you do at work?

Did you have any special training?

What special memories do you have of work days?

Did you do National Service?

Adulthood

Do/did you have a partner?
Partner's name/occupation?

Where and when did you meet?

Where and when did you marry?

What did you wear? What flowers did you have?

Where did you go on honey-moon?

Where did you live?

Any children – what are their names?

Any grandchildren – what are their names?

Did you have any special friends? What are their names?

When and where did you meet? Are you still in touch?

Did you have any pets? What were their names?

Retirement

When did you retire?

What were you looking forward to most?

What were your hobbies and interests?

What were the biggest changes for you?

Likes and dislikes

What do you enjoy doing now?

What do you like to read?

What is your favourite colour?

What kind of music do you like?

What are your favourite foods and drinks?

Is there anything that you definitely do not like to do?

How you like to do things

Do you have any special routines to your day?

What time do you like to get up in the morning? And go to bed at night?

Do you want people to help you with anything?

Do you want people to leave you to do anything on your own?

How do you like people to address you?

What are you good at?

Is there anything else you would like to tell us about you?

Pool Activity Level (PAL) Checklist

Name: Date: Outcome:

Completing the Checklist: for each activity, the statements refer to a different level of ability. Thinking of the last two weeks, tick the statement that represents the person's ability in each activity. There should be only one tick for each activity. If in doubt about which statement to tick, choose the level of ability that represents their average performance over the last two weeks. Make sure you tick one statement for each of the activities.

1. Bathing/Washing

- Can bathe/wash independently, sometimes with a little help to start   P: ☐

- Needs soap put on flannel and one-step-at-a-time directions to wash   E: ☐

- Mainly relies on others but will wipe own face and hands if encouraged   S: ☐

- Totally dependent and needs full assistance to wash or bathe   R: ☐

2. Getting dressed

- Plans what to wear, selects own clothing from cupboards; dresses in correct order   P: ☐

- Needs help to plan what to wear but recognises items and how to wear them; needs help with order of dressing E: ☐

- Needs help to plan, and with order of, dressing, but can carry out small activities if someone directs each step S: ☐

- Totally dependent on someone to plan, sequence and complete dressing; may move limbs to assist   R: ☐

3. Eating

- Eats independently and appropriately using the correct cutlery   P: ☐

- Eats using a spoon and/or needs food to be cut up into small pieces   E: ☐

- Only uses fingers to eat food   S: ☐

- Relies on others to be fed   R: ☐

4. Contact with others

- Initiates social contact and responds to the needs of others   P: ☐

- Aware of others and will seek interaction, but may be more concerned with own needs   E: ☐

- Aware of others but waits for others to make the first social contact   S: ☐

- May not show an awareness of the presence of others unless in direct physical contact   R: ☐

5. Groupwork skills

- Engages with others in a group activity, can take turns with the activity/tools   P: ☐

- Occasionally engages with others in a group, moving in and out of the group at whim   E: ☐

- Aware of others in the group and will work alongside others although tends to focus on own activity   S: ☐

- Does not show awareness of others in the group unless close one-to-one attention is experienced   R: ☐

6. Communication skills

- Is aware of appropriate interaction, can chat coherently and is able use complex language skills   P: ☐

- Body language may be inappropriate and may not always be coherent, but can use simple language skills   E: ☐

- Responses to verbal interaction may be mainly through body language; comprehension is limited   S: ☐

- Can only respond to direct physical contact from others through touch, eye contact or facial expression   R: ☐

7. Practical activities (craft, domestic chores, gardening)

- Can plan to carry out an activity, hold the goal in mind and work through a familiar sequence; may need help solving problems   P: ☐

- More interested in the making or doing than in the end result, needs prompting to remember purpose, can get distracted   E: ☐

- Activities need to broken down and presented one step at a time; multisensory stimulation can help to hold the attention   S: ☐

- Unable to 'do' activities, but responds to the close contact of others and experiencing physical sensations   R: ☐

8. Use of objects

- Plans to use and looks for objects that are not visible; may struggle if objects are not in usual/familiar places (i.e. toiletries in a cupboard below washbasin   P: ☐

- Selects objects appropriately only if in view (i.e. toiletries on a shelf next to washbasin)   E: ☐

- Randomly uses objects as chances upon them; may use inappropriately   S: ☐

- May grip objects when placed in the hand but will not attempt to use them   R: ☐

9. Looking at a newspaper/magazine

- Comprehends and shows interest in the content,
  turns the pages and looks at headlines and pictures   P: ☐

- Turns the pages randomly, only attending to items pointed
  out by others   E: ☐

- Will hold and may feel the paper, but will not turn the
  pages unless directed and will not show interest in the content   S: ☐

- May grip the paper if it is placed in the hand but may not
  be able to release grip; or may not take hold of the paper   R: ☐

Select the appropriate PAL Profile to act as a general guide to engaging with the person in a variety of activities.

Complete a PAL Individual Action Plan to act as a specific guide to facilitating personal activities.

	Planned	Exploratory	Sensory	Reflex
TOTAL				

Pool Activity Level (PAL) Profile

Name: **Date:**

Planned Activity Level

Likely abilities

Can explore different ways of carrying out an activity

Can work towards completing an activity with a tangible result

Can look in obvious places for any equipment

Likely limitations

May not be able to solve problems that arise

May not be able to understand complex sentences

May not search beyond the usual places for equipment

Method of engagement

Activity objectives	To enable ………… to take control of the activity and to master the steps involved
Position of objects	Ensure that equipment and materials are in their usual, familiar places
Verbal directions	Explain activities using short sentences, avoiding connecting phrases such as 'and', 'but', 'therefore', or 'if'
Demonstrated directions	Show ………… how to avoid possible errors
Working with others	…………… is able to make the first contact and should be encouraged to initiate social contact
Activity characteristics	There is a goal or end product, with a set process, or 'recipe', to achieve it. An element of competition with others is motivating

Suitable activities (based on knowledge of the person's life history)

....

....

Pool Activity Level (PAL) Profile

Name: **Date:**

Exploratory Activity Level

Likely abilities   **Likely limitations**

Can carry out very familiar activities   May not have an end result in
in familiar surroundings   mind when starts an activity

Enjoys the experience of doing an   May not recognise when the
activity more than the end result   activity is completed

Can carry out more complex   Relies on cues such as diaries,
activities if they are broken down   newspaper, lists and labels
into two-to-three step stages

Method of engagement

Activity objectives	To enable .... to experience the sensation of doing the activity rather than focusing on the end result
Position of objects	Ensure that equipment and materials are in the line of vision
Verbal directions	Explain activities using short simple sentences. Avoid using connecting phrases such as 'and', 'but', 'therefore', or 'if'
Demonstrated directions	Break the activity into two-to-three steps at a time
Working with others	Others must approach .... and make the first contact
Activity characteristics	There is no pressure to perform to a set of rules, or to achieve an end result. There is an element of creativity and spontaneity

Suitable activities (based on knowledge of the person's life history)

....

....

Pool Activity Level (PAL) Profile

Name: **Date:**

Sensory Activity Level

Likely abilities

Is likely to be responding to bodily sensations

Can be guided to carry out single-step activities

Can carry out more complex activities if they are broken down into one step at a time

Likely limitations

May not have any conscious plan to carry out a movement to achieve a particular end result

May be relying on others to make social contact

Relies on cues such as diaries, newspaper, lists and labels

Method of engagement

Activity objectives

To enable ………… to experience the effect of the activity on the senses

Position of objects

Ensure that ………… becomes aware of equipment and materials by making bodily contact

Verbal directions

Limit requests to carry out actions to the naming of actions and objects, e.g. 'Lift your arm', 'Hold the brush'

Demonstrated directions

Show ………… the action on the object. Break the activity down into one step at a time

Working with others

Others must approach ………… and make the first contact. Use touch and …………'s name to sustain the social contact

Activity characteristics

The activity is used as an opportunity for a sensory experience. This may be multisensory and repetitive

Suitable activities (based on knowledge of the person's life history)

....

....

Pool Activity Level (PAL) Profile

Name: **Date:**

Reflex Activity Level

Likely abilities   **Likely limitations**

Can make reflex responses to   May be in a subliminal or subcon-
direct sensory stimulation   scious state

Can increase awareness of self,   May have difficulty organising the
and others, by engagement of   multiple sensations that are being
senses   experienced

May respond to social engage-   May become agitated in an envi-
ment through the use of body lan-   ronment that is over-stimulating
guage

Method of engagement

Activity objectives	To arouse ………… to a conscious awareness of self
Position of objects	Stimulate area of body being targeted, e.g. stroke …………'s arm before placing it in a sleeve
Verbal directions	Limit spoken directions to movement directions, i.e. 'Lift', 'Hold', 'Open'
Demonstrated directions	Guide movements by touching the relevant body part
Working with others	Maintain eye contact, make maximum use of facial expression, gestures and body posture for a nonverbal conversation. Use social actions which can be imitated, e.g. smiling, waving, shaking hands
Activity characteristics	The activity is in response to direct selective sensory stimulation

Suitable activities (based on knowledge of the person's life history)

....

....

Pool Activity Level (PAL) Individual Action Plan

Name: **Date:**

Dressing

Favourite garments
Preferred routine
Grooming likes and dislikes

Method:

Bathing

Favourite toiletries
Preferred routine
Bathing likes and dislikes

Method:

Dining

Favourite foods
Preferred routine
Dining likes and dislikes

Method:

Pool Activity Level (PAL)
Individual Action Plan Guidance Notes

Refer to the level of ability for each activity that has been revealed on the **PAL Checklist** and enter the methods for facilitating the engagement of the person with cognitive disability onto the relevant section of the **Individual Action Plan**.

Activity: Dressing

Planned Activity Level

- Encourage (the person) to plan what to wear and to select own clothes from the wardrobe.

- Encourage (the person) to put on (his/her) own clothes; be available to assist if required.

- Point out labels on clothing to help orientate the back from the front.

- Encourage (the person) to attend to grooming such as brushing hair, putting on make-up, cleaning shoes.

Exploratory Activity Level

- Encourage discussion about the clothing to be worn for the day: is it suitable for the weather or the occasion? Is it a favourite item?

- Spend time colour-matching items of clothing and select accessories.

- Break down the activities into manageable chunks: help lay the clothes out in order so that underclothing is at the top of the pile. If the person wishes to be helped, talk (the person) through the activity: 'Put on your underclothes'; 'Now put on your dress and cardigan.'

- Encourage (the person) to check (his/her) appearance in the mirror.

Sensory Activity Level

- Offer a simple choice of clothing to be worn.

- Spend a few moments enjoying the sensations of the clothing: feeling the fabric, rubbing the person's finger up and down a zip fastener, or smelling the clean laundry.

- Break down the activity into one step at a time: 'Put on your vest'; 'Now put on your pants'; 'Now put on your stockings'; 'Now put on your dress.'

Reflex Activity Level

- Prepare the clothing for (the person), ensure the dressing area is private and that a chair or bed at the right height is available for sitting.

- Talk through each stage of the activity as you put the clothing onto (the person). Use a calm tone, speak slowly and smile to indicate that you are nonthreatening.

- Stimulate a response in the limb being dressed by using firm but gentle stroking. Ask (the person) to assist you when necessary by using one-word requests: 'Lift'; 'Stand'; 'Sit'.

- At the end of dressing, spend some time brushing (the person's) hair using firm massaging brush strokes.

Activity: Bathing

Planned Activity Level

- Encourage (the person) to plan when they will have the bath, to draw the water and select toiletries from the usual cupboard or shelf.

- Encourage (the person) to wash (his/her) own body; be available to assist if required.

- Encourage (the person) to release the water afterwards and to wipe the bath.

Exploratory Activity Level

- Break down the activity into manageable chunks: suggest that (the person) fills the bath, then when that is accomplished suggest that he or she gathers together items such as soap, shampoo, flannel, and towels.

- When (the person) is in the bath, suggest that (he/she) soaps and rinses (his/her) upper body and, when that is accomplished, suggest that (he/she) soaps and rinses (his/her) lower body.

- Ensure that bathing items are on view and that containers are clearly labelled.

- Have attractive objects around the bath (such as unusual bath oil bottles or shells) and encourage discussion and exploration of them.

Sensory Activity Level

- Prepare the bathroom and run the bath water for (the person).

- Make the bathroom warm and inviting – play music, use scented oils or bubble bath, have candles lit on a safely out-of-reach shelf.

- Break down the activity into one step at a time and give (the person) simple directions: 'Rub the soap on the cloth, rub your arm, rinse your arm, rub your chest, rinse your chest...'

Reflex Activity Level

- Prepare the bathroom and run the bath water for (the person), put in scented bath products (lavender will aid relaxation).

- Ensure that the bathroom is warm and inviting, and feels secure by closing the door and curtains and providing a slip-resistant bath mat in the bath and on the floor. Clear away any unnecessary items that may be confusing.

- Use firm, massaging movements when soaping and rinsing (the person). Wrap (him/her) securely in a towel when (he/she) is out of the bath.

Activity: Dining

Planned Activity Level

- Encourage (the person) to select when and what (he/she) wishes to eat.

- Encourage (the person) to prepare the dining table and to select the cutlery, crockery and condiments from the usual cupboards or drawers.

- Encourage (the person) to clear away afterwards.

Exploratory Activity Level

- Store cutlery and crockery in view and encourage (the person) to select his or her own tools for dining.

- Offer food using simple choices.

- Create a social atmosphere by using table decorations, music and so on, promoting conversation.

Sensory Activity Level

- Serve food so that it presents a variety of colours, tastes and textures.

- Offer (the person) finger foods; encourage (him/her) to feel the food.

- Offer (the person) a spoon, place it in (his/her hand) and direct (him/her) to 'Scoop the potato'; 'Lift your arm'; 'Open your mouth' and so on.

Reflex Activity Level

- Use touch on (the person's) forearm to make contact, maintain eye contact, and smile to indicate the pleasure of the activity.

- Place a spoon in (the person's) hand. Close your hand over (the person's) and raise the spoon with food on it to (his/her) mouth.

- As the food reaches (the person's) mouth say 'Open' and open your own mouth to demonstrate. Try stroking (the person's) cheek gently as you offer the food.

The Pool Activity Level (PAL) Outcome Sheet

Name:						
Activity:						
Date:	/ /	/ /	/ /	/ /	/ /	/ /

LEVEL OF ENGAGEMENT 0 = never, 1 = sometimes, 2 = always

COGNITIVE ABILITIES						
Goal-aware						
Motivated						
Attention to detail						
Concentrates						
Appears interested						
Responds to sensations						
Explores objects						
PHYSICAL ABILITIES						
Standing/mobile						
Seated						
Uses tools						
Co-ordinated						
Grips objects						
Releases objects						
SOCIAL INTERACTION						
Aware of others						
Starts conversations						
Makes vocal noises						
Responds to others						
Aware of needs of others						
Shares in the group activity						
Makes eye contact						
WELL-BEING						
Shows enjoyment						
Shows humour						
Assertive						
Makes choices						
Bored						
Angry						
Frightened						
Anxious						
Restless						
Sleepy						
TOTAL ENGAGEMENT SCORE						

Part 2 – Using the Pool Activity Level (PAL) Instrument in Leisure Activities

Sarah Mould and Jackie Pool

Chapter 10

Introduction to Part 2

Engaging people in meaningful activities provides the opportunity for them to think, feel and do – it is this that is proven to be essential to physical and mental health. Activities that have meaning for people, which excite their interest and also enable them to use a range of skills, optimise their potential for well-being.

As care givers for people who have cognitive impairments caused by, for example, dementia, stroke or learning disability, we are all gifted with the opportunity and possibility that engaging a person in an activity can provide.

In order to understand the importance of the opportunity for activity, it is helpful to consider the model of 'Emotional Need' described by Tom Kitwood (1997, pp.80–84). An understanding of the elements of this model often has an extremely profound impact on care givers, not only in terms of what it is to be a human being, but what it must be like to live with a cognitive impairment.

Kitwood's 'Emotional Needs' model describes six elements:

- *love* being the core

- attachment

- comfort

- identity

- inclusion

- **occupation**.

Care givers realise the importance of all of these elements, including 'occupation' but somehow the words 'tasks', 'activities', 'achievement' and 'skills' can evolve into 'lack of time', 'too few staff', 'no resources', 'not part of my job', 'not valued', 'not trained'.

Care givers need support from their team leaders and managers to become 'reflective practitioners', who consistently demonstrate the following type of outlook:

- We can enable a person to get dressed rather than 'get' a person dressed.

- Simply engaging in conversation with a person is undertaking an activity.

- Reading through a daily newspaper *with* the person being cared for is a valuable occupation.

- Playing a game of cards or facilitating some creative work with a person can be carried out without fear of chastisement because the laundry has not been put away.

Obstacles described by many care givers are the lack of resources or equipment to carry out an activity and lack of guidance as to how to facilitate successful activities. Not all care homes have access to occupational therapy services or the resources to employ activity co-ordinators. Indeed, one might observe that this is part of the cause of the problem – do we need to rely on 'designated' people to undertake activities with service users?

The Pool Activity Level (PAL) Instrument Profile will help care givers to understand the needs and skills of individuals in order to facilitate the right activity at the right time and at the right level. Once this is understood perhaps care givers will have increased motivation and enthusiasm to facilitate meaningful engagement in personal care activity, domestic activity and in leisure activity. Many care givers have hobbies and interests that have helped them to develop a range of skills that they can bring to the workplace. Is that support worker who is focusing on making beds and finishing the laundry may also be a skilled artist? Is that care worker who 'gets ten people up and dressed in two hours' also a dab hand at card games?

People with cognitive impairments may have difficulty engaging in such activities, particularly if the activity is too demanding or not presented to the person in an understandable way. Care staff trying to provide leisure activity programmes can be at a loss to know how to offer the activity to maximise success, or how to find equipment locally or nationally.

Part 2 of this edition of the PAL book has therefore been developed to guide care givers to improve their skills when facilitating leisure activities. Ideas for four Activity Packs are set out in the next four chapters. A selection of possible activities to be included is listed for each pack. This is not an exhaustive list and care givers may choose to omit some and to add others. Possible sources for the activities are identified at the end of the book, but care givers may choose to search other means of obtaining them.

Each chapter includes guidance on carrying out a range of activities with individuals who have different levels of ability, as revealed by the completion of the PAL Instrument Checklist. The four Activity Packs are:

- table-top games activities

- social games activities

- creative activities

- sensory activities.

REFERENCE

Kitwood, T. (1997) *Dementia Reconsidered: The Person Comes First.* Buckingham: Open University Press.

Chapter 11

Table-top Games Activities Pack

SUGGESTED CONTENTS

- Large-print Scrabble
- Large-piece jigsaw (x2)
- Large-print playing cards
- Large-size playing cards
- The game 'Frustration'
- Large-piece dominoes
- Card holder (for four)

INTRODUCTION

This pack will be appropriate for those who have been established as having ability at either the **planned** or **exploratory** level using the Pool Activity Level (PAL) Instrument.

The activities within this pack can be used with a single person or a small group. The number of people involved in each activity will be determined by the type of activity, skills and abilities of the participants, environment/room available and care staff available to facilitate.

Guidance regarding the number of people to engage with each activity is given. The length of time the activity lasts will be determined by the response of the individuals and will rely upon the facilitator's observational skills to determine when the activity should cease.

People with moderate to severe cognitive impairments may have a very short attention span and the activity may only be appropriate for a few minutes. One of the benefits of some of the activities in this pack is that they do not need to be put away when someone has finished using them. Where possible, the activity can be left out so that the person can return to it when he or she feels like engaging with it again. This opportunity for spontaneity is extremely valuable when working with people with cognitive impairments.

UNDERSTANDING THE ABILITY OF THE PERSON

Understanding what the person can and cannot do is vital to the success of the activity. If the activity is too difficult, a person may become anxious or frustrated. If the activity is too easy, the person may feel unmotivated to take part.

The activities within this pack are likely to be very familiar to people. However, it is essential that care staff understand at which level the individual is functioning in order that the right amount of support and facilitation can be offered and the activity be presented in the right way.

All of the activities within this pack require myriad cognitive skills: attention and concentration, problem solving, memory and planning, as well as awareness of rules, visual and symbolic recognition, numerical and word-finding skills and fine motor dexterity.

The ways in which people with cognitive impairments are supported to undertake and enjoy these activities will hinge on the skill, understanding and knowledge of the care staff.

Never allow yourself to find that you are playing *for* the person rather than *with* the person.

PLANNED ACTIVITY LEVEL

At a **planned** activity level the person can work towards completing a activity but may not be able to solve any problems that arise while in the process. He or she will be able to look in obvious places for equipment needed but may not be able to search beyond the usual places. A care giver assisting someone at this level will need to keep his or her sentences short and avoid using words like 'and' or 'but', which tend to be used to link two sentences together into a more complex one. Care givers will also need to stand by to help solve any problems should they arise. People functioning at a planned activity level are able to carry out activities that achieve a tangible result.

EXPLORATORY ACTIVITY LEVEL

At an **exploratory** activity level the person can carry out very familiar activities in familiar surroundings. However, at this level people are more concerned with the effect of doing the activity than in the consequence and may not have an end result in mind. Therefore a creative and spontaneous approach by care givers to activities is helpful. If an activity involves more than two or three activities, a person at this level will need help in breaking the activity into manageable chunks. Directions need to be made very simple and the use of memory aids such as activity lists, calendars and labelling of frequently used items can be very helpful.

LARGE-PRINT SCRABBLE

Scrabble is a word game for two, three or four players. Play consists of forming interlocking words, crossword fashion, on the Scrabble playing board, using letter tiles with various score values. The objective of the game is to get the highest score.

Each player competes by using their tile combinations and locations that take best advantage of letter values and premium squares on the board. There is a very thorough instructions booklet with the game, which care staff are advised to read and have to hand when playing.

In this large-print edition the letters on the tiles are enlarged to enable players with cognitive impairments to have the maximum opportunity for visual recognition and thence letter identification. Of course, players may also have a visual impairment, so the enlarged letters will be equally valuable.

You will know which of the people you provide care for are likely to enjoy Scrabble.

Consider the person's:

- personality – do they enjoy word games or crosswords?

- biography – has the person always been interested in language and vocabulary. Are they a past 'Scrabble champion'? Did they play the game with their friends and family?

- cognitive ability – what is the person's attention span; do they recognise words and letters; do they have a vocabulary of words within their memory; could they solve problems?

- social factors – do they enjoy company; are there people to whom they seem to relate well and who have similar interests; are they aware of social rules such as turn taking; are they easily distracted?

- physical factors – does the person have the fine motor skills to manipulate the letter tiles?

These and many more facets of the person need to be considered when inviting the person to play Scrabble so that it is made as rewarding and enjoyable an experience as possible.

When playing with a person at the **planned** level, be conscious of how you present the game. Ask if they have played it or seen it before. People at this activity level may have difficulty in grasping the instructions if they are described in full. Break the instructions down, e.g. 'This is the playing board'; 'These are the letters. I'll put them in this bag. Please take seven (count them out with the person). Put them on this rack' and so on.

Constantly gauge the person's response to the activity and level of instruction and adapt your approach as required.

People at the **planned** level will have difficulty in solving problems as they arise. Ask them if they would allow you to help them and suggest to them what they might do. Leave the decision up to the person – it may not be the decision that you would have made. (Remember: you are playing *with* them not *for* them.)

Sometimes people with cognitive impairments may have word-finding difficulties and may create words. Be advised by the game rules and the other players as to whether a word is acceptable or not. Although some debate is healthy, argument is not to be encouraged and you may need to mediate.

People who are at the **planned** level will be looking for an outcome: an end product to the activity in terms of a winner. Gauge how long to play the game in order that the participants have an opportunity to identify a winner, end the game and be congratulated on their performance.

When playing with people at the **exploratory** level, be mindful that the end result will not be as important to them. They may enjoy examining the tiles and the textures of the game components. Instructions, again, must be very simple and will require repetition.

You may consider the person at this level working as part of a team with a member of care staff to provide support and to help maintain the focus required.

Be prepared for and welcome spontaneity. Certain words may elicit reminiscence or recitation of song or poetry – welcome this.

As facilitators you must use all your skills to observe the response of the participants, adapt your approach if required, offer help if requested and maintain the momentum of the activity but at the participant's pace. It may be helpful to set a time to play to and identify the winner at that point. However, people at an **exploratory** level of ability may not be as concerned with the end result of winning as with the enjoyment in taking part.

Upon completion of the game, thank everyone for joining in. They may want to assist you to put the Scrabble away. (As there are many small components to the game, it is not advisable to leave it out.)

LARGE-PIECE JIGSAW

Working on a jigsaw puzzle has long been associated with peaceful contemplation and relaxation. (There may be occasional outbursts of frustration too!) Some may consider jigsaw puzzles a childish pursuit, but look in any hobby store and you will find myriad jigsaws surrounded by adults who enjoy the fascination of completion and vibrancy of the picture.

Completing a jigsaw can be a solitary pursuit if that is someone's preference or can be an opportunity for a pair to engage in true teamwork as one mind.

The jigsaw puzzles suggested for this Activity Pack are composed of large pieces but have pictures that are appropriate for adults. They are designed to enable people to achieve success through maximising opportunities for visual recognition, problem solving and manipulation among other cognitive skills. The large pieces are also helpful if people have difficulty with fine motor skills.

Again, your knowledge of the person will indicate whether a jigsaw puzzle would be a suitable activity. However, if someone shows an interest but has never done a jigsaw before, do not preclude them from taking part – they may have discovered a new pastime.

Ascertain that the person would like to complete a jigsaw. Consider the person's:

- personality – do they enjoy puzzles?

- biography – has the person always been interested in table-top games?

- cognitive ability – what is the person's attention span; do they recognise colour and shapes; can they solve problems?

- social factors – do they enjoy company; are there people to whom they seem to relate well and who have similar interests; are they aware of social rules such as turn taking, or would they prefer to complete a jigsaw alone?

- physical factors – does the person have the fine motor skills to manipulate the pieces?

If people are at the **planned** level, they may prefer to be left alone to complete the jigsaw independently. (Make sure they do not find it so easy as to feel patronised.)

If the people are at the **exploratory** level, ask if they would permit you to help them. Clearly if they would prefer to do it themselves, encourage them. In both cases maintain a position where you will be available for help if needed.

You may like to set the jigsaw up so that it can be left out after the person has finished with it, either completed or uncompleted. This will maximise the opportunity for spontaneity; the person can place a piece almost as they walk by or become engaged with it for a longer period.

You may wish to consider purchasing a variety of jigsaw puzzles to suit the different needs and abilities of the people you care for. It would be useful to have a range of pictures that relate to different individuals' interests.

PLAYING CARDS AND CARD HOLDERS

Card games are very familiar to a wide range of people and have been a source of enjoyment for centuries. The appearance of a pack of cards, the colours, suits, design and shape are recognised by people throughout the world. People with cognitive impairment are likely to recognise a pack of cards by using their visual recognition skills and memory; possibly they have been a life-long card player, either as a solitary pursuit or in a team, at a bridge club, or the casino, or perhaps a game of cards was a regular activity within the home or in the pub.

Not everyone will enjoy playing cards, and for some it might be objectionable because of religious or cultural beliefs. As with all activities, it is essential to use your knowledge of the person before offering an activity.

Two sets of playing cards are suggested within this pack: a regular-size pack of cards with large print and a large-size pack of cards.

When engaging a person in a game of cards you need to consider the person's:

- personality – is this something that they show an interest in? Have they initiated the idea of playing cards? (You may wish to consider having the packs of cards in view, perhaps on a table or cupboard to enable individuals to find them and perhaps instigate a game.)

- biography – do they have prior experience of playing cards?

- cognitive ability – are they able to engage in a game independently or will they require assistance to maintain the rules of play and to problem solve?

- social factors – do they enjoy company; are there people to whom they seem to relate well and who have similar interests; are they aware of social rules such as turn taking? Would they prefer games for one person, such as Patience? Are they easily distracted?

- physical factors – do they have the fine motor skills to manipulate the cards and the larger movement ability to reach across a card table?

People at a **planned** activity level are likely to be able to engage in a game independently if the game is familiar to them and they have a good attention span. You may consider the following card games:

- Pontoon or 21s

- Black Jack

- Rummy

- Canasta

- Poker

- Patience

- Bridge.

If a person with cognitive impairment could teach the game to a care giver this would be a highly motivating and enriching experience for the person. You may wish to consider if a care giver needs to be involved. Perhaps a person could be set up with a game of Patience to engage with on his or her own. If it is possible to leave the card game out, the person can leave and come back to it if he or she chooses.

A care giver need not be involved at all. If you are in a residential home or day service, you could introduce residents or service users to each other in order that they could share their enthusiasm for card games. There should be a quiet area where a game of cards can be played. Consider the environment carefully to minimise distractions associated with noise, poor lighting and interruptions.

The regular pack of cards has large print, which will maximise the opportunity for a person with visual impairment or difficulty with visual recognition to participate in a game.

Card holders are also recommended for this pack because they are of benefit to people who have difficulty holding a hand of cards. You can also place the hand of cards in a card holder to enable the person to see each card more easily.

The large pack of cards enhances this even further, though you may wish to use this pack in a different way. People at the **exploratory** activity level may enjoy a team game based on the television programme 'Play Your Cards Right.'

1. You will need a method whereby you can place the large playing cards upright. (If you have a flipchart you can place the cards in the groove at the bottom so that they lean against the board. If you have a fairly narrow piece of furniture, you could place the cards on this so that they lean against the wall. Otherwise you could place the cards flat on a table but make sure everyone can see them.)

2. Shuffle the cards and place six of them face down so that the back of the cards is showing.

3. Identify a quiz master and two teams.

4. Ask each team in turn a quiz question.

5. If they get the question right they can move on to the six cards prepared.

6. Turn the first card over. Advise the team that they need to decide whether the next card will be higher or lower than this card.

7. If the team correctly predicts whether the card will be higher or lower, allocate 10 points and move on to the next card.

8. If the team correctly predicts all six cards allocate them an extra 100 points.

9. Clear this row of cards and replace with six new ones, placed face down.

10. Move on to the next team and repeat the process.

11. The winning team is the one with the highest score after all the playing cards have been used.

Game rules

- If the first card turned over is the same as the first card in the line, the team can choose to change it.

- If, further down the line, the card is the same as the previous one, the team has lost as it is neither higher nor lower than the previous card. (You may wish to use the catchphrase 'You get nothing for a pair…not in this game!' as Bruce Forsyth did in the game show.)

- If the team incorrectly predict the turn of the card, the other team can take over and try to complete the line. If they make an error, pass back to the other team.

- Do not use the jokers. Aces are high (higher than the king).

Try to get into the spirit of the game (this will be very easy), with lots of 'oohs' and 'aahs' at the turn of the cards to increase the anticipation and tension.

You could use the large cards to play Patience but you will need a very large table!

If you would like to invest in a second pack of large playing cards you could use this to play Pairs. Sort the cards from both packs into pairs. Lay these randomly on a table face down, no more than eight pairs. The person with cognitive impairment is asked to turn a card over and identify it. Then turn over a second card. If they match, remove both from the table. If they do not match, turn both over, face down, and continue. The game is over when all cards are paired.

Or you could play the perennial favourite Snap. Each player has a pack of cards and places them on the table in front of them face down. In turn, place a card face up on the table. If the cards match, the first person to shout 'Snap!' wins the whole stack of cards. The winner is the person who ends up with all the cards.

The response of the individuals playing will determine how long the game of cards will last. Remember that people with cognitive impairment may have a short attention span, so one game may be enough.

Do not correct the actions the person takes if they choose to do something that you may not have done. Use tact, verbal suggestion and shared problem solving to support someone who is making errors that appear to be affecting their sense of well-being and enjoyment.

Monitor for signs of confusion, disinterest or distraction and adapt your approach accordingly. The objective of the game is enjoyment and a sense of achievement. Again, do not patronise people by taking over or playing for them, and make sure that the level is correct for each individual so that they do not find the game too hard or too easy.

Thank the participants for joining in the game and allow some time for reflection.

You may like to consider setting up a 'Cards Club' as a regular weekly event if appropriate.

THE GAME 'FRUSTRATION'

Board games are a popular pastime in homes and clubs throughout the world. Competition, problem solving and fun are all key components in participating in a board game.

The game Frustration which is suggested in this pack makes use of several cognitive functions and is therefore suited to people at the **planned** and **exploratory** levels. Because the dice is enclosed within the board it is also less likely to be lost.

The amount of support and guidance required will vary according to the activity level of the person and their skills and interests. It is important, in a pastime such as this, that you do not mix participants from different activity levels.

At a **planned** level, the participants are likely to require ongoing reminding of the rules of play and guidance perhaps as to what to do for each move, as they are likely to have difficulty with problem solving. Participants at this level may be quite competitive. Therefore it is important that they do not feel 'held back' by someone who is at a different activity level and who may not be able to respond as quickly or who does not maintain interest throughout.

At an **exploratory** level, the participants are likely to be less concerned with the outcome of the game, more interested in taking part and the process. Again, it is likely that the participants will require verbal and gestural prompting to maintain their focus on the game and to be able to sequence each step effectively. Therefore it is important that they are not playing with someone at a different activity level as they may be responded to in a negative way if they do not maintain the pace of the game or make 'mistakes'.

The game has detailed instructions of play on the back of the box. Take time to read through and understand them, so that as a facilitator you can maintain the focus and momentum of the activity. (Have the instructions next to you just in case!)

Consider the person's:

- personality – is this something that they show an interest in?

- biography – do they have prior experience of playing this game or other similar games such as Ludo?

- cognitive ability – is the person able to engage in a game independently or will they require assistance to maintain the rules of play and to problem solve? Can the person recognise colour? They will need to be able to do so in order to distinguish between the four colours used in the game.

- social factors – do they enjoy company; are there people to whom they seem to relate well and who have similar interests; are they aware of social rules such as turn taking; are they easily distracted?

- physical factors – does the person have the movement skills and strength to push the dice shaker and the larger movement ability to reach across the board? (It may be appropriate to consider teams of pairs – one participant and one care giver per team to support each other in cognitive and physical process needs.)

Upon completion of the game, thank everyone for joining in and allow time for reflection. The participants may wish to help you put the game away.

LARGE-PIECE DOMINOES

The large-piece dominoes that you will include in this pack are suited to the needs of people with cognitive and sensory impairment. The size of the dominoes ensures that maximum opportunity is provided for people with visual, numerical and symbolic recognition difficulties to participate in this pastime. The dominoes are suitable for people with visual impairment, the black dots on the pale background making identification quite easy. People with manual dexterity problems will also find the large-size dominoes easier to manipulate.

The instructions for play are usually included in the dominoes box and are easy to follow.

You will have a good understanding of the skills and interests of the person with cognitive impairment in order to know whether the person would enjoy a game of dominoes and at what level to present the activity.

A game of dominoes is an excellent activity for promoting social interaction too, providing an opportunity for engagement between players. They may have reminiscences of playing dominoes before or may like to share stories of pastimes they have enjoyed. Encourage this.

At the **planned** activity level, it is likely that the person will be able to participate in the activity independently by playing with one other person or a group of people. The person may require occasional prompting with the placing of the dominoes. Offer assistance when requested, and do not be intrusive. For example, if someone is having difficulty locating or choosing a domino ask if the person would allow you to look at the dominoes and facilitate the decision-making process in choosing a domino. Let the person place the domino on the table. *Do not* do this for the person unless he or she asks you to. Offer positive reinforcement throughout the activity.

At the **exploratory** activity level, the person may need more support and facilitation with identification of the domino and knowing where to place it on the table. Again, do not be intrusive. You may like to consider playing the game in pairs to enhance focus and enjoyment based on feelings of agency and success.

Let the response of the participants guide you as to how long to play. The whole experience should be relaxing and enjoyable for all, so make sure that you play in an environment as free from distraction as possible.

Thank the players for participating in the activity and allow some time for reflection.

Chapter 12

Social Games Activities Pack

SUGGESTED CONTENTS

- Parachute
- Ring-toss set
- Sing-along tape and song book
- Skittles set
- Bean-bag target

INTRODUCTION

This pack will be appropriate for those who have been established as having ability at either the **planned**, **exploratory** or **sensory** level using the Pool Activity Level (PAL) Instrument.

As the title of this pack would suggest, the activities contained are intended to be used with a group of people. The number of people within the group will be determined by the type of activity, skills and abilities of the participants, environment/room available and care staff available to facilitate. Guidance as to numbers for each activity is given within this chapter.

The length of time the activity lasts will be determined by the response of the individuals and will rely upon the facilitator's observational skills to determine when the activity should cease. Though these are group activities it is essential that each individual's response is monitored to observe signs of well-being and ill-being.

Some of these activities are quite physical so facilitators need to be aware of individuals' stamina, mobility and physical health needs. Be aware too that people with moderate to severe cognitive impairment may have a very short attention span.

UNDERSTANDING THE ABILITY OF THE PERSON

Understanding what the person can and cannot do is vital to the success of the activity. If the activity is too difficult, a person may become anxious or frustrated. If the activity is too easy, the person may feel unmotivated to take part. The nature of these activities also requires that people engage with others socially. People do not respond well when they feel pressured to take part in an activity when they do not wish to. Some people may feel uncomfortable or embarrassed in front of other people. Some may not be used to the company of others. Of course, some people thrive on social contact and all the positive reinforcement this can bring. People with moderate to severe cognitive impairment may not be aware of 'social norms' and rules. This will therefore require facilitators to observe the group dynamics and adjust the activity if required to ensure that the aims of the activities are achieved.

PLANNED ACTIVITY LEVEL

At a **planned** activity level the person can work towards completing a activity but may not be able to solve any problems that arise while in the process. He or she will be able to look in obvious places for equipment needed but may not be able to search beyond the usual places. A care giver assisting someone at this level will need to keep his or her sentences short and avoid using words like 'and' or 'but', which tend to be used to link two sentences together into a more complex one. Care givers will also need to stand by to help solve any problems should they arise. People functioning at a **planned** activity level are able to carry out activities that achieve a tangible result.

EXPLORATORY ACTIVITY LEVEL

At an **exploratory** activity level the person can carry out very familiar activities in familiar surroundings. However, at this level people are more concerned with the effect of doing the activity than in the consequence and may not have an end result in mind. Therefore a creative and spontaneous approach by care givers to activities is helpful. If an activity involves more than two or three activities, a person at this level will need help in breaking the activity into manageable chunks. Directions need to be made very simple and the use of memory aids such as activity lists, calendars and labelling of frequently used items can be very helpful.

SENSORY ACTIVITY LEVEL

At a **sensory** activity level the person may not have many thoughts or ideas about carrying out an activity: he or she is mainly concerned with the sensation and with moving his or her body in response to those sensations. People at this level can be guided to carry out single-step activities such as sweeping or winding wool. More complex activities can only be carried out when directed one step at a time. Therefore care givers need to ensure that the person at this activity level has the opportunity to experience a wide variety of sensations and to carry out one-step activities. Directions to maximise this opportunity need to be kept very simple and to be reinforced by demonstrating the action required.

PARACHUTE

The word 'exercise' often conjures up images of going to the gym or jogging – not always possible, appropriate or desired. However, participation in physical exercise is essential to maintain health and well-being. Evidence shows that participation in exercise has psychological benefits too. It can also be fun!

A parachute as a means of exercise and social engagement may not have been your first consideration. However, for people at both **exploratory** and **sensory** activity levels, this entirely suits their need to enjoy the process of an activity that has simple, straightforward steps and sensory input.

Why a parachute?

- Parachute activity promotes co-operation. Everyone shares the same equipment at the same time, so working together rather than against each other is the aim. The parachute naturally forms a circle, so everyone will form around this and be able to see each other, enhancing awareness of others.

- There are no losers in parachute games.

- Parachute games are flexible in terms of the amount of time used and opportunities for spontaneity. The parachute is lightweight and, once unfurled, ready to use.

- Parachutes lend themselves to the imagination. This may be the first time that someone has even seen a parachute, let alone worked with one. This rare sight can therefore trigger the creative senses.

- The facilitator/s actively participate too.

One is never too old to play, but consideration must be given to older people with cognitive impairment who may require this activity to be presented in a different way.

Understanding the ability of the person

Consider the person's:

- personality – do they enjoy social gatherings and physical activity?

- biography – have they handled a parachute before? (Be prepared for some reminiscence about this before the activity begins.)

- cognitive ability – are they able to maintain attention and sustain their hold of the parachute?

- social factors – do they enjoy company; are there people to whom they seem to relate well?

- physical factors – are they in a wheelchair? Do they have respiratory or cardiac problems, arthritis or any inflammatory disease, tender skin, osteoporosis or have they recently suffered a bone injury; do they have difficulty with balance and co-ordination as a result of a stroke or neurological impairment?

It may not be possible to undertake parachute games outdoors, therefore consideration of the environment is essential. There should be space for six to eight people to form a circle in the room. The ceiling height should be sufficient for the parachute activities and the needs of people who use wheelchairs should be considered.

Suggested session plan

You may wish to spend some time exploring the parachute with the group before you begin the games.

1. Explain to the group that you have a parachute. Remove it from the bag and allow it to spread out over the floor. It may be appropriate for all the group participants to be seated in stable, straight-backed chairs.

2. Allow each of the participants to feel the texture of the parachute by placing some of the material on their lap and encouraging them to touch and hold it. Monitor each person's response. If the person shows signs of distress or disinterest or requests not to join in, allow the person to leave the group and enable the person to choose whether he or she would like to sit and watch or do something else individually.

3. If the remainder of the group are willing, support each individual to hold one or two of the handles. Consider the number of facilitators required and where they are placed in terms of providing the optimum amount of support to individuals.

4. Begin by encouraging the participants to slowly lift their arms up and down until the parachute is inflating and deflating rhythmically. Play some appropriate music in the background to encourage pace and to set mood. Constantly monitor the response of the individuals. There can be quite a draught when the parachute deflates. Also be aware of any expressions of pain or stiffness.

5. Allow the group to rest the parachute on their laps, still holding on to it.

6. Facilitate the group to pass the parachute round – still keeping it spread out, encouraging hold and release of the parachute handles. Pass it back the other way. Check for responses. It is hoped that there will be laughter, verbal and nonverbal communication. Mirror these responses.

7. Facilitate the group to raise and lower their arms alternately as quickly as they are able, to give a ripple effect to the parachute.

8. Follow this again with gentle raising and lowering of arms as in step 1.

9. Allow the group to rest for a few moments. Ask how they are feeling and check that they are happy to continue.

10. Facilitate the group to lift and lower their arms again. Inform them that you are going to throw a very light ball onto the parachute and that their activity is not to let it fall off. As the parachute inflates throw a light, brightly coloured ball onto the parachute (helpful if it's a contrasting colour). Encourage the group to use their hand–eye co-ordination to lift their bit of the parachute to keep the ball on it. Check for responses and over-exuberance, which can be quite frightening and offputting for some people.

If the group is happy to continue you might like to try one of the games described below. The more familiar you become with the games, the more likely that you will be able to adapt this plan according to the needs and preferences of your group members.

Other activities you might like to try

'Mushroom'

Everyone holds the parachute taut. On the count of three, everyone lifts the parachute high above their heads. A giant mushroom is formed. Encourage the participants to watch as the parachute slowly descends.

(If you have enough space or are using the parachute outside you could play the 'Floating Mushroom' by facilitating the group to let go of the parachute when it is fully lifted above their heads.)

'Igloo'

This is a game for people standing or in wheelchairs. Lift the parachute high above the heads like a mushroom. Take a couple of steps in, or assist the person in the wheelchair by pushing them forward, and bring the parachute down behind you with everyone facing each other inside.

'Parachute golf'

Invite the participants to hold the parachute fairly taut. The facilitator throws a ball or several balls into the parachute with the instruction that the participants work together to get the balls to go through the hole in the middle of the parachute. (Make sure the balls are smaller than the hole in the parachute!)

Make sure that you end the group by approaching each individual in turn and thank them for joining in. Take the parachute from them and begin to roll the parachute up in readiness for putting away. Spend a few moments of quiet reflection together or play some relaxing music to enable the participants to feel calm and relaxed and to return the heart rates to normal!

RING-TOSS SET

Many people are familiar with the game 'Hoop La'. This next activity may therefore have some familiar associations for the participants.

If necessary, prepare the target before you invite people to join in a game. This activity can be played with any number of people but it is recommended that there are no more than six to eight in the group. It becomes increasingly difficult for people with cognitive impairment to maintain focus and interest in an activity if they are not engaged for most of the time. Waiting for other people to take their turn in an activity can be frustrating and boring for some, who may then leave the activity either cognitively or physically.

Understanding the ability of the person

Consider the person's:

- personality – do they enjoy social gatherings and physical activity?

- biography – have they played similar games before? (Some people may relate this to childhood and may not wish to play a 'childish' game – this should be respected.)

- cognitive ability – are they able to maintain attention and sustain their participation in the competition?

- social factors – do they enjoy company; are there people to whom they seem to relate well?

- physical factors – are they in a wheelchair? Do they have respiratory or cardiac problems, arthritis or any inflammatory disease, osteoporosis or have they recently suffered a bone injury; do they have difficulty with balance and co-ordination as a result of a stroke or neurological impairment? You will need to ensure that the participants have fairly good manual dexterity, balance and visual skills. It may be more beneficial for the participants to play this game sitting down.

Arrange the group in a circle of comfortable chairs and place the target in the middle of the floor within the circle. Use your judgement and knowledge of the participants to gauge how far the target needs to be from them.

This is a competitive game, but be mindful of facilitating each individual within the group to experience success, no matter what their ability. You can facilitate the game as a group of individuals but it is much more fun, and more sociable, to facilitate the group in teams. You can ask each team to give themselves a name, which will emphasise identity and place participants in a mutually co-operative situation of support.

Demonstrate how the game is played and agree any rules with the participants such as the number of rounds, whether the target can be moved, when to have a break or refreshments, etc. You will need a score board.

Toss a coin to decide which team will begin. Begin Round 1.

The first player in the team is handed the rings and facilitated to throw them toward the target, aiming to achieve a high score by getting the rings over the dowels. At the **planned** level you may need to verbally encourage the person to do this; at an **exploratory** level you may need to physically demonstrate a throwing action; and at a **sensory** level you may need to guide the person to make a throwing action by placing your hand over theirs.

Record their score and move on to the first player in the next team. Ensure that each player in each team has a go. Record the combined total of all the players as the team score. Move on to Round 2.

At the end of the game, total the scores for each round and announce the winning team.

Ensure that throughout the game you are offering lots of encouragement through verbal and nonverbal reinforcement for each individual as they take their turn.

Remember that for people at the **planned** level it is possible that they will be quite competitive among themselves as individuals and within their teams. This will help to maintain focus for the participants, but they may require assistance to problem solve if anything 'unplanned' happens. At the **exploratory** level, the action of throwing the rings and involvement in the social camaraderie of the activity is likely to be more fulfilling than the end result of the game. For those at the **sensory** level, the sensation of the rings in their hands, the action of throwing, the audible enjoyment of the activity will be stimulating.

Thank the group for their participation. Put the ring-toss equipment to one side.

You may wish to end the session with some relaxing music, allowing the participants to chat quietly and reflect on the session.

SING-ALONG TAPE AND SONG BOOK

'Singing is an invigorating activity which usually promotes a happy feeling, provides a means of releasing tensions and is often evocative of past experiences and emotions.'

(Mercer, F. (2006) *Song Book – Words for 100 Popular Songs*. Winslow Press)

As part of everyday life, music is more than just a noise, and often holds personal significance. The Sing-along Tape and Song Book can be presented to people at the **planned** level and **exploratory** level in the same way.

Understanding the ability of the person

Consider the person's:

- personality – what type of music do they enjoy? Music is a very personal choice. One person's delight may be another's racket, so selecting the 'right' songs while catering for a range of tastes is important.

- biography – it is likely that some of the songs may provoke recall and reminiscence of earlier days and experiences. This is extremely useful in terms of engagement and communication. Be mindful of strong emotion, which may be expressed in tears – of joy or sorrow. Be prepared to support individuals in the expression of these emotions, being aware that they are among others.

- cognitive ability – do they have difficulty with speech? It is often found that people with profound verbal language impairment may still be able to sing fluently. Can they recognise the words on the song sheet? If the song is familiar this may not matter as the words may come back to them when they hear the music

- social factors – are they comfortable singing in a group, do they prefer just to listen or are they a 'performer'?

- physical factors – do they have a hearing impairment; do they need to wear a hearing aid; do they need to be positioned closely to the speaker or someone with a strong singing voice to enable them to hear? Do they have a visual impairment? The Song Book is in large print but may need to be made larger for some participants.

When organising a sing-along, explain to the individuals what is going to happen and verify that they are happy to participate. Seat the group in comfortable chairs, preferably in a circle so that everyone can see each other and feel included.

You will have decided which songs you are going to use and have set the tape or CD up so that it will begin at the correct place.

If you decide to make photocopies from the book please refer to the copyright regulations at the front of the Song Book regarding reproduction. (Your organisation can contact the Copyright Licensing Agency Ltd on 020 7631 5555 for advice about fees.)

Tell the group the name of the first song they will be singing. Ensure that everyone is prepared and start the tape.

The facilitator/s have a key role in encouraging the group to sing and should always feel comfortable to start the singing and ensure that the group members are singing too, by using facial expression and hand gestures such as conducting.

Sing the first song, all the while monitoring the response of the participants to ensure that they feel comfortable. Participants must not be forced to join in with the singing; listening is an equally important activity. At the end of the song, pause the tape and ask the group if they enjoyed it. If the group is happy to, continue with the next song. Gauge continuously the response of the participants. Some may spontaneously stand and dance – encourage this if safe to do so.

When all the songs have been sung, the participants might like to choose a song to sing again. Again, be mindful of the responses of the group. If a participant appears distressed, offer reassurance but do not assume that they want to leave the group; check with them.

Thank everyone for joining in. Consider suggesting a regular 'sing-along' and agree when to meet again. Play some gentle music to enable the participants to relax, or by gauging the response of the group play the tape again, or another well-known musical tape, allowing the participants to join in spontaneously.

People at a **sensory** level may like to listen to the songs. It is unlikely that they will follow the words from the book, but they may sing spontaneously, or hum. They may also enjoy using some musical instruments such as tambourines or maracas to play along to the music.

SKITTLES SET

As a social pastime, many people participate in bowling, either at a skittles alley or on the bowling green. Bowling is an enjoyable activity and, by its very nature, a social one.

A bowling set can be utilised by people who are functioning at the **planned**, **exploratory** or **sensory** level.

The number of people you engage in this activity will be determined by their interests, preferences and physical abilities. You will also need a lot of space and a smooth floor of wood, lino or close-weave carpet.

Understanding the ability of the person

Consider the person's:

- personality – do they enjoy social gatherings and physical activity?

- biography – have they played bowls before; perhaps they have belonged to a club?

- cognitive ability – are they able to maintain attention on the game and to follow the rules? Can they let go of the bowling ball to roll it towards the skittles or the jack?

- social factors – do they enjoy company; are there people to whom they seem to relate well?

- physical factors – are they in a wheelchair? Do they have respiratory or cardiac problems, arthritis or any inflammatory disease, osteoporosis or have they recently suffered a bone injury; do they have difficulty with balance and co-ordination as a result of a stroke or neurological impairment?

In order to set up the activity, ensure that the area is hazard free and that you have lots of room for people to move around.

Set up the skittles in a triangular formation, one skittle at the front, then two placed behind adjacent to each other, then three in a line at the back. Decide how far the distance between the bowler and the skittles will be and place a marker of some kind to indicate where the bowler will stand. This will form your 'bowling alley'.

Place a row of chairs either side of the alley facing each other. This will be where your teams will sit. The distance between the chairs will be determined by the physical needs of the participants.

You will need a scoreboard to record each individual's score and thence team score which will be totalled at the end. There may be a person who does not want to be involved in the bowling, but who would enjoy being the score master.

Introduce the activity to the participants and demonstrate what they need to do (to bowl each of the balls in turn in an attempt to knock down as many skittles as possible).

Facilitate the participants to form teams and encourage them to name their team. Toss a coin to identify which team will start. Encourage the first player on the team to bowl. Record their score and then request the first player of the next team bowls and so on. The amount of support each individual will need will depend upon the activity level they are within and their physical abilities. You can bowl sitting down, but good trunk control and balance are needed. A chair with arms will be helpful, and if it is needed the person should be encouraged to hold onto the arm with the 'nonbowling' hand.

Make sure you give lots of verbal and nonverbal reinforcement of each individual's achievement – urging the ball on, cheering when a skittle is hit, groaning when a skittle does not fall, shouting 'strike' if all the skittles are knocked down at once.

Monitor the response of the individuals for signs of poor attention, lack of interest or distress. This will gauge the pace of the activity and when to end it.

People at the **planned** level will enjoy the competitive nature of the game. At the **exploratory** level people will enjoy the process of the game, the running of the ball, and the response of their team members. At the **sensory** level, you may need to offer the participants hand-over-hand support to facilitate holding and release of the ball. The distance between the bowler and skittles will need to be minimal to ensure success and maximum sensory input.

At the end of the activity, thank everyone for participating. Allow for quiet conversation between the participants and encourage them to reflect on the activity.

BEAN-BAG TARGET

This activity can be used to promote the use of physical, social and cognitive skills.

For people who are within the **planned**, **exploratory** or **sensory** levels, this activity can be adapted to suit their skills and abilities.

Understanding the ability of the person

Consider the person's:

- personality – do they enjoy social gatherings and physical activity?

- biography – have they played similar games before?

- cognitive ability – are they able to maintain attention on the game and to follow the rules? Can they let go of the bean bags as they throw them?

- social factors – do they enjoy company; are there people to whom they seem to relate well?

- physical factors – are they in a wheelchair? Do they have difficulty with balance and co-ordination as a result of a stroke or neurological impairment? Do they have arthritis in the joints of their hands that may affect their ability to grip the bean bag?

To play this as a straightforward physical game, unwrap the target and lay it out on a smooth floor, target side up. The pack may already come with bean bags; you may choose to use all or some of them depending on the skills and abilities of the participants. You may purchase bean bags separately and then make your own target. You will need a scoreboard.

The aim of the game is to achieve as high a score as possible by throwing the bean bags one at a time onto the target. The more toward the centre the bean bag lands, the higher the score. If a bean bag lands on the line between two numbers, count the score that the majority of the bean bag is on. (Referee's decision is final!)

You may wish to facilitate this activity for a group of four to six individuals. Or you may like to facilitate as a team game, following the guidelines for the ring-toss activity. The person or team that attains the highest score is the winner.

For participants at the **planned** level, you can introduce an additional component to the game which will enable participants to use their cognitive skills too. As individuals or within a team, facilitate the activity as described above. After each individual turn, a score is achieved. You can then offer the participants the opportunity to 'double their score' by answering a quiz question. If they answer correctly the double score is achieved and recorded on the scoreboard. If they answer incorrectly, the original score is recorded.

Your knowledge of the participants will determine the difficulty of the questions asked: too difficult and the participants may feel disheartened, losing interest and attention; too easy and the participants may feel that they are being made fools of and again lose interest.

An additional element can be introduced by asking the participants to choose a category they want to answer a question on, e.g. 'food & drink', 'entertainment', 'geography', etc.

There is a wide variety of quiz books available in book shops, some based on well-known television quizzes, which you may consider a valuable resource when undertaking activities.

For participants at the **exploratory level**, the satisfaction will be in the process of the game. Your knowledge of each individual will determine whether you include the quiz element to the game.

Your explanation of the activity will need to be clear and broken down into small steps, perhaps prompting each participant by giving them one bean bag at a time while verbally encouraging and physically demonstrating the throw.

For participants at the **sensory** level, the enjoyment of the game will be in the texture of the bean bags in their hands, the sound of the bags hitting the target, the vocalisations of the participants. You may need to offer hand-over-hand support to facilitate hold and release of the bean bags.

At all levels, be mindful of the distance of the target from the participants, giving consideration to their physical skills and needs. For people at a **planned** level, the target could be some distance. For those at the **exploratory** level, the target may need to be closer. For those at a **sensory** level, the target may need to be closer still.

Throughout the game, the facilitation style must be enthusiastic and encouraging. Give lots of verbal and nonverbal feedback and encourage the participants to engage with each other and use their communication skills.

The duration of the game will be guided by the response of the participants. As it finishes, thank everyone for joining in and allow them to sit quietly for a while to reflect and relax.

Chapter 13

Creative Activities Pack

SUGGESTED CONTENTS

- A3 coloured paper
- Paint brushes
- Paint disc set
- Felt-tip pens
- PVA glue
- Collage assortment pack
- Modelling dough
- Modelling set
- Glass pens
- Glass painting cards

INTRODUCTION

Humans have endeavoured to leave their mark on the world since prehistoric times, when the walls of caves were used to record the activities and practices of mankind at that time. Since then art has been the conduit for the expression of one's creative self, the glorification of gods and rulers, the recording of historical events, for capturing memories, for pleasure and for the innate need to communicate through colour, light and shape.

Whether a professional or amateur artist, the satisfaction upon completion of something one has created cannot be underestimated, nor can the sense of achievement at the response and recognition of others toward the piece of work.

Art is so much more than simply 'putting brush to paper'. The ideas in this Activity Pack are designed to be used to develop and guide you in facilitating people with cognitive impairments to undertake art/creative activities. You will not be providing art therapy for your clients/service users. In order to offer art therapy you need to have completed many years of training. (Indeed it can be dangerous to attempt to use any therapy techniques unless you have been trained to do so.)

The activities described in this section are designed to be used with people at the **planned**, **exploratory** and **sensory** activity levels.

You will have a good understanding of who is likely to enjoy participating in a creative activity through knowledge of their personality, biography and response to such activities. Do not preclude people who have not undertaken creative activities in the past. This may have been more due to circumstances than choice. Continue to consider people who have a lot of experience in creative arts, indeed may have been involved professionally. However, be aware of their current skills and abilities compared to what they may have been in the past. Do not place people in an activity which may reinforce their lost skills. Think about presenting creative activities in a different way but always according to their activity level.

KNOW THE ACTIVITY

You do not have to be a trained artist to be able to facilitate an art or craft activity. However, an interest in this type of activity is essential in order to enthuse and engage the participants fully. This book provides you with some ideas as to the sort of activities you may like to facilitate.

You must be sure that you know what the process of the activity is so that you can assist with problem solving and maintain the focus of the activity. Ensure that you have fully prepared for the activity, that you have all the equipment to hand, and that any co-facilitators understand what is expected of them.

There is a vast range of books and videos available that may be worth investing in.

It may be worth investigating whether your local craft store offers classes in particular art or craft activities for facilitators to develop ideas and skills. Perhaps consider a local evening class for yourself and for the person with cognitive impairment. You might also like to consider arranging for an artist or art teacher to offer some classes to facilitators and people with cognitive impairment. Sometimes local art colleges provide sessional input, particularly if it is made part of a student assignment.

(Don't forget about the application of health and safety policies, including the protection of vulnerable adults and the principles of confidentiality if you do engage people from outside your organisation.)

KNOW THE ENVIRONMENT

The facilities and equipment required will obviously depend on the particular activity. A designated area with table and chairs is ideal, although some settings may prefer to use the dining room between meals. The key is that it can be easily cleaned and has access to a sink and water.

Secure storage must be provided for sharp and potentially dangerous tools, as well as toxic materials such as adhesives. There should be relevant completed risk assessments associated with the use and storage of toxic or dangerous materials. Good ventilation, lighting and temperature are essential.

It is extremely important that there is quiet and privacy available to enable participants to fully engage. Distraction and interruption will hinder the ability to focus and concentrate. Nobody likes drawing or painting with an audience behind them!

This pack will be appropriate for those who have been established as having ability at either the **planned**, **exploratory** or **sensory** level using the Pool Activity Level (PAL) Instrument

Most of the activities in this pack can be undertaken with an individual on his or her own or in a small group. Guidance as to the recommended number of participants is given throughout this chapter. Knowledge of the individual, his or her level of ability, skills, interests, personality and biography will act as the primary guide for care givers as to whether to present a creative activity to the individual.

The length of time each activity lasts will be determined by the type of activity and, primarily, by the individual's response to the activity. This relies on the care giver's observational skills to determine when the activity should cease. People with moderate to severe cognitive impairments may have a very short attention span and the activity may only be appropriate for a very short while.

If safe to do so, some of the activities could be left out for the individual/s to return to when they feel ready. Guidance is given as to the type of activity which could be left out, but a risk assessment for each activity may need to be completed according to the needs of the individuals, the environment and type of service.

UNDERSTANDING THE ABILITY OF THE PERSON

Understanding what a person can and cannot do is vital to the success of the activity. If the activity is too difficult, a person may become anxious or frustrated. If the activity is too easy, the person may feel unmotivated to take part.

Engaging in art and craft activities can provide not only a feeling of personal satisfaction and relaxation during the activity, but also a sense of achievement and lasting pleasure in the end result.

Of course, art and craft activities are not everyone's 'cup of tea'. Occasionally people may associate some of the activities with school days and be hesitant to engage, according to whether they felt they were 'good at art' or not.

It is also essential that people are not placed in a position where they become aware that they are not as skilled as they used to be in a creative activity as this can be devastating and lead to the person declining to participate at all.

Consideration at all times must be given to the person's previous experience of creative activities. It is not recommended that someone who was an accomplished artist is given a 'paint by numbers' to complete. This can be very demeaning and negate the skills and life experience of the person. Neither would you ask someone who has no experience of creative activities to undertake a complex craft activity or still-life drawing.

This does not mean that these people cannot be facilitated to engage in a creative activity, however. It is essential that you have a clear understanding of the activity level of the person so that you know how to present the activity and what sort of activity to offer.

The same issues may need to be considered for the care givers who will be facilitating a creative activity. Again, some facilitators may have a natural aptitude for creative activities; indeed, it may be a regular pastime for them. Other care givers may not feel at all confident or interested in creative activities. Ensure that their skills are identified and used in other activities.

Make the most of the 'creative' people in your team; use their skills and ideas.

POTENTIAL BENEFITS OF CREATIVE ACTIVITIES

- May revive a familiar hobby/interest.
- May facilitate learning of a new skill or interest.
- Can improve hand dexterity and co-ordination.
- Stimulates the senses.
- Facilitates decision-making skills.
- Stimulates the imagination.
- Enables people to experience a sense of achievement.
- Facilitates communication.
- Facilitates reminiscence and orientation.
- Can place someone in the role of expert.

PLANNED ACTIVITY LEVEL

At a **planned** activity level the person can work towards completing a activity but may not be able to solve any problems that arise while in the process. He or she will be able to look in obvious places for equipment needed but may not be able to search beyond the usual places. A care giver assisting someone at this level will need to keep his or her sentences short and avoid using words like 'and' or 'but' which tend to link two sentences together into a more complex one. Care givers will also need to stand by to help solve any problems should they arise. People functioning at a **planned** activity level are able to carry out activities that achieve a tangible result.

EXPLORATORY ACTIVITY LEVEL

At an **exploratory** activity level the person can carry out very familiar activities in familiar surroundings. However, at this level people are more concerned with the effect of doing the activity than in the consequences and may not have an end result in mind. Therefore a creative and spontaneous approach by care givers to activities is helpful. If an activity involves more than two or three activities, a person at this level will need help in breaking the activity into manageable chunks. Directions need to be made very simple and the use of memory aids such as activity lists, calendars and labelling of frequently used items can be very helpful.

SENSORY ACTIVITY LEVEL

At a **sensory** activity level the person may not have many thoughts or ideas about carrying out an activity; he or she is mainly concerned with the sensation and with moving his or her body in response to those sensations. People at this level can be guided to carry out single-step activities such as sweeping or winding wool. More complex activities can only be carried out when directed one step at a time. Therefore care givers need to ensure that the person at this activity level has the opportunity to experience a wide variety of sensations and to carry out one-step activities. Directions to maximise this opportunity need to be kept very simple and to be reinforced by demonstrating the action required.

UNDERSTANDING THE ABILITY OF THE PERSON

Consider the person's:

- personality – are they motivated to take part; are they interested in art/craft? Do they have an awareness that their level of skill in this activity may not be as good as it was? This will have a huge effect on their sense of self and confidence. How will they view the activity? You will need to ensure that you present it in an appropriate manner so that participants do not feel that the activity is childish or that they are being treated like children. Would they be active or passive during the activity?

- biography – do they have good memories of this activity that will enhance their confidence and self-esteem or do they have negative memories associated with this activity that may be painful for them?

- cognitive ability – do you know for how long each person is able to concentrate? Do they require very specific, simple, one-step instructions to be able to participate? Do they understand what is being asked of them? Do they comprehend the purpose of the activity or are they more likely to enjoy the sensation of the activity? Are they able to solve problems if required? Do they have intact visual-recognition skills for all the equipment used? Are they able to use their memory to remember familiar skills and actions? Are they able to express their preferences, choices and wishes? Do they have a sense of control over their environment and activities and opportunities?

- social factors – do they enjoy company; are there people to whom they seem to relate well? Are they able to express their emotions? Art may be a useful technique for expression in the absence of words. Would the person prefer to engage in the activity on his or her own or in a small group? What is their preferred communication method; do they use a variety of communication techniques, verbal and nonverbal, or do they have difficulties with communication? Do they enjoy being with others; are they able to understand functions such as sharing and turn taking?

- physical factors – are they able to sit for the duration of an activity; do they require their seating to be at a certain height; are they able to tolerate sitting in a straight-backed firm chair? Do they have a good range of movement; are they able to reach items required; can they utilise all of the paper or does it need to be made smaller? Do they have good dexterity and co-ordination; can they hold a paint brush or pencil; would they benefit from an adaptation to the brush or pencil? Do they have arthritic pain, stiffness to the joints? Do they have a neurological impairment affecting their physical ability such as a tremor requiring support or a weakness to one side of their body or a paralysis? (An occupational therapist will be able to advise you on how to enable and support people with these difficulties to participate in an art activity.)

What are the sensory needs of the person?

Does the person have a visual impairment; can they see strong, primary colours and pattern? Does the person wear glasses and are these clean? Can they see the edge of the paper or card; is there a contrasting colour underneath? Does the person have a hearing impairment; do they need to be able to hear instructions or to participate in the activity? Do they wear a hearing aid; is it switched on? Is the person able to use their other senses, e.g. touch for craft-type activities, texture and shape, using hands as a paint brush? Could you enhance the experience of the person by engaging their sense of smell, perhaps by using very aromatic flowers, spices or fruits?

GLASS PAINTING CARDS AND GLASS PENS

Cards are available in a range of themes, including Christmas, Easter, birthdays or anniversaries. This activity will be extremely useful in providing assistive cues in orientating the person with cognitive impairment to the time of year.

The sending of Christmas cards, for example, has been an essential part of the celebration of Christmas since Victorian times. Many people are likely to have a strong memory for this activity and may recall the feelings associated with the giving and receiving of cards.

It is equally likely that people will have some experience of making greetings cards – either as a child or adult, or in helping children to make cards. There is an understanding, too, that receiving a handmade card is something extra special in recognition of the thought, time and effort put into this.

People who enjoy art and craft will enjoy this activity because it involves elements of both pastimes.

The activity of glass painting cards is designed to be carried out with people at the **planned** and **exploratory** levels.

Packs vary depending on the source but typically consist of:

- card templates

- acetates, each with pictures etched onto them

- glass pens/markers.

Instructions for completing a card

1. Choose a picture and cut along outer edge (where indicated) to remove from sheet.

2. Using glass pens, colour in the picture, remaining within the black lines.

3. Choose a card and remove detachable outer edge and detachable oblong of card where the picture will go.

4. Fold the card at indentation.

5. Remove the white tissue backing from the picture on the acetate.

6. Carefully place the picture behind the oblong hole on the front of the card. Ensure that the coloured surface is facing outward.

7. Using double-sided clear tape, or glue which dries clear, attach the picture to the inside of the card.

8. You may like to use some glitter or glitter pens to decorate the outer edge of the card.

Presentation of this activity to a person at the planned activity level

A person at the **planned** activity level will very much enjoy this activity in terms of working towards a tangible end result. The steps for completion of the greetings card are clearly defined and very straightforward and the person is likely to require minimum prompting to complete each step. Though the steps for completion of the card are defined, there is room for personal creativity in terms of choice of the picture and colours used to complete it and choice of card to stick the picture in.

When facilitating a person to engage in this activity, it may be a good idea to have a completed card to show in order to enable the person to envisage what the end result will be and what can be achieved. (The 'here's one I made earlier' technique is very useful.)

Be mindful that the pictures are simple and may be construed as being quite 'childish'. People may associate the idea of 'colouring in' as a childhood pursuit. However, people can be encouraged to participate in terms of the simplicity of the cards; the process of 'colouring in' can be very relaxing and provide stimulation for the senses. This activity also promotes choice and decision-making skills.

A group of people at the **planned** activity level may wish to engage in this activity together, either as a group of individuals or as a team. Perhaps forming a production line where different steps in the process are undertaken by different people would be fun: one person cutting out the pictures, one or two colouring them, one sticking them on the card, one or two people decorating the cards, etc. Make sure that you provide an opportunity for everyone to undertake each step of the activity at some point. This will be highly motivating for the participants who will be using not only their creative and cognitive skills, but also their communication and social skills.

The activity also assists a person at the **planned** level as all the equipment needed is in front of them; they do not need to search for it.

Facilitators for this activity need to ensure that they fully prepare and organise the activity in advance.

- Identify an area where there will be no distractions or interruptions if possible.

- Ensure that the room is well lit and that the temperature is appropriate. There will need to be a source of ventilation as the glass pens smell strong.

- Prepare the table and ensure that all the equipment you need is there.

- Make sure there are enough comfortable seats for everyone.

- Be prepared to offer advice, support and prompting as required.

- Give praise and reinforcement throughout.

- Consider what is to be done with the completed cards. Will the participants keep them? Could they be sold, if appropriate, as contribution to the service's funds? Involve the participants in this decision.

Presentation of this activity to a person at the exploratory activity level

A person at the **exploratory** level will enjoy this activity because of its familiarity and opportunity to be creative. People at this activity level will enjoy the process of the craft, the stimulation of the senses and the opportunity for social engagement. They are likely to be less concerned with the end result.

You can use the same techniques for engaging, preparing and facilitating as detailed above. Be mindful of the skills and abilities of each individual in terms of dexterity, attention and concentration, problem solving. They may require more intense support and guidance from facilitators to enable them to remain focused and to gain a sense of pleasure and achievement.

Accuracy may not be as important as the taking part for this group of individuals; therefore be careful that you do not refer to errors in a negative way or attempt to correct errors unless requested to, as this will impact on the participants' sense of well-being and motivation to participate.

Collaboration of participants and facilitators in this activity is essential and great fun!

Upon completion of this activity thank all the participants for their contribution and for joining in. Allow time for reflection, perhaps by looking at the completed cards and talking about them, favourite colours, designs, etc. Encourage participants to reminisce about the season; perhaps enjoy a cup of tea together while doing so. Some participants may like to assist you in clearing up after the activity.

Additional ideas

If participants have enjoyed this activity, they may like to continue glass painting as a club. Glass paints and pens are readily available from most craft shops and some stationers. You could save and collect a store of jam jars and glass bottles for people to paint. You will need a black glass marker to draw the design on the glass first. Enable participants to be spontaneous and creative using abstract and representational designs.

You could also try painting on glass sheets. The process is quite simple. Encourage participants to choose a picture, perhaps from a magazine, and trace over it with tracing paper using a black felt-tip pen. Place the tracing under a sheet of A4 glass. Using a glass pen or marker, follow the tracing underneath so that the picture is replicated onto the glass. Remove the tracing paper from underneath. Colour the drawing in using glass paints or pens. Consider framing the pictures by placing a piece of black card behind the finished picture and installing in a suitable frame.

People may like to paint their own designs directly onto the glass.

WARNING

Glass pens and markers are spirit based. Ensure that these are not ingested and are used in a well-ventilated room. They may stain skin and clothes.

REFER TO MANUFACTURER FOR GUIDANCE.

Be cautious in the use of glass to guard against breakage and possible cuts.

You may consider undertaking a risk assessment of the activity and individuals to inform you as to how to proceed or reduce the risks identified.

ART/CREATIVE ACTIVITIES USING PAPER, PAINT AND FELT-TIP PENS
For people at the planned activity level

A regular 'art' group, perhaps once a week, may be of great interest and very motivating for people. You can decide the theme of each session together in advance. The group members may wish to concentrate on their own work or participate in a group piece. Suggested themes:

- still-life work, e.g. fruit, vegetables, interesting objects, flowers

- architecture and buildings

- landscape

- self-portrait

- people

- animals

- the seasons

- view from a window.

Be mindful of different levels of artistic ability within the group, particularly if you are sharing the work. Some people may wish to keep their work private. Respect this. You may consider working from photographs or pictures. Facilitate this by reinforcing the link between the photo and the painting or drawing to enable participants to remain focused. Make sure the photo is big enough for them to see.

Consult with the participants about what they wish to be done with the completed work. Are there opportunities for framing work? Would the group consider an art exhibition once or twice a year?

Greetings cards

It may be possible that people will enjoy using their art work to make greetings cards. You may need to frame their work in strong card so that it is more substantial. Again, craft shops have an array of pictures, printing tools, transfers and materials specifically for card making.

Imagination

Make use of a person's imagination, playfulness and creativity. Encourage participants to paint from their imagination or perhaps a cherished memory. Facilitate this process by writing down the person's ideas so that he or she is assisted to recall and maintain focus on the picture.

Abstract designs

The paint and paper could also be used for printing a design or abstract. Ensure that the person's clothing is protected. Have a variety of fruits, vegetables, leaves, flowers suitable for printing with, for example, half an apple, piece of carrot cut crossways, oak leaf – anything hard (that will withstand paint and pressure) and with an interesting design. Cover the surface to be printed in paint and place down firmly on paper for a few seconds. Carefully lift the object off. Repeat. Allow the prints to dry. These can be used as background for other pieces of work if desired.

Use the paper and paint, pens, etc., for abstract work, emphasising pattern, design and flow of ideas. This may be a difficult concept for some participants who may be more conscious of concrete ideas, 'recognisable' art. It may be useful to have ideas and pictures for them to see and perhaps copy using a colour of their choice.

Creative writing

Rather than using the paper and pens for drawing, consider using them for creative writing. This is particularly good in a small group. Agree what you would like to write about. Enable the participants to choose colours and write their ideas, according to the topic, on the paper. This may be a little daunting for some participants, so a better idea is for the facilitator to write down what the group say according to the topic and colour choices. This takes great concentration by the facilitator, who must write down what the participants say, not their interpretation of what is said.

Suggested topics:

- the seasons, using colour to represent each of the different seasons

- the weather, again using colour to represent the different types, e.g. 'It was a beautiful summer's day (orange). The sun shone brightly (yellow)…'

- holidays, using colour to represent different countries, beaches, etc.

- special occasions

- the countryside.

Some people may like to complete their own piece of writing or use a combination of picture and writing to express a particular theme or idea.

For people at the exploratory activity level

This group of people are likely to enjoy the process of the activity, being less concerned with the end result. They will enjoy the opportunity to use and explore colours, shapes and designs. With some encouragement they may be stimulated by the other members of the group and engage in conversation about what they are doing or what it reminds them of. People at the exploratory activity level may not be able to concentrate for too long at a time, so consider artistic activities that have fairly quick results.

Simple scenes

Participants may enjoy completing a skyscape or a seascape. This can be achieved quite quickly by using broad, sweeping strokes with the paint brush loaded with paint across the paper. The participants may require guidance as to the choice of colours, perhaps blues and greens for sea and sky, reds and yellows for sunset. Have some examples or photographs to inspire them.

Painting to music

This is a very enjoyable and relaxing activity. You will need to prepare a variety of musical styles, but may wish to concentrate on relaxing tunes: the classics or 'chilled' CDs available from shops. Inform the participants that they will be using their imagination and allowing their arm and the paint brush or pen to move as though it is 'dancing to the music'. Play some music to engage the attention and then ask the participants to paint or draw whatever comes to mind or just to move their arm across the paper in time to the music. You may need to use demonstration for this activity. There may be a variety of results: representational and abstract.

String painting

You may like to engage the participants in another kind of printing technique. Fold a piece of paper in half. Dip a long piece of string in paint and lay it over one half of the paper in a random design. Close the other half of the paper over it and press down hard. If there is an end of the piece of string hanging out between the folded paper, pull it out *without* opening the paper. Once the string is removed, open the paper to see the results!

N.B. Any kind of technique that has an element of surprise will be very motivating and engaging for people at the **exploratory** (and **sensory**) activity level. Another idea is to again fold a piece of paper in half. On one side of the paper use lots of paint to make an abstract design; the design should touch the fold of the paper but not go over it. When the person is satisfied with the design, fold the paper in half over the design and press gently. *Do not* rub the design as this will result in a mucky splodge! Carefully unfold the paper and admire the results.

These techniques are somewhat messy. Be guided by the response of the participants as to whether they feel comfortable with this. Ensure that clothing is protected.

Art corner

Do not underestimate the artistic skills of people at the **exploratory** activity level. Encourage people to use these skills by setting up an 'art corner' for them or ensuring that there are art materials readily available to them, to make use of moments of spontaneity.

People at this activity level will also enjoy creative writing, particularly if they do not need to do the writing! This is a marvellous opportunity for social interaction and reminiscence, recorded for posterity, and a chance to be creative with words. The fact that it is being recorded on a large piece of paper and in full Technicolor will enable the participants to maintain focus on the activity and enjoy the process.

For people at the sensory activity level

You may wish to facilitate someone in a one-to-one art activity to enable the person to experience as much sensory stimulation as possible.

A person at the **sensory** level will not be concerned with the outcome of the activity or necessarily the process. What they will enjoy is the colour, shapes, textures, and sounds which you can introduce into an art activity.

The individual activities do not have to last a long time; a fairly immediate result will be very motivating for the individual whose concentration skills may be quite limited.

Guided colouring

The person may respond to stark, contrast images of no more than two colours. Having a pre-drawn outline on a large piece of paper for the person to paint is one idea. The outline could be of a face in silhouette or an animal or familiar object. You will need to guide the person, perhaps using hand over hand, to dip a large, thick brush into the paint and place it on the paper. Use broad sweeping strokes to enable the person to experience the sensation of movement.

You can use the same idea for painting flowers. Use a whole piece of paper and a black pen to draw a huge flower (not too complex). Facilitate the person to paint the petals, leaves and stem in colours of their choice. Use any object or theme of particular interest or relevance to the person.

Be mindful of visual impairment and cognitive impairment. The person's world may be quite small to him or her so you may wish to try this technique on a piece of A4 paper to enable the person to focus on it a little easier.

Again, the outcome is not of importance here. It is the person's sensory experience of the activity that is important.

Hand painting

Some people may enjoy a very simple printing technique – brushing paint over the hand, placing it firmly on paper and removing it to reveal a print. Feet are sometimes fun to print with too.

If you are hoping to engage a person at the **sensory** level in this activity, be very mindful of the potential risks and comfort of the person. Your knowledge of the person will enable you to decide whether this would be enjoyable for the person. By constantly monitoring their verbal and nonverbal response, you will know whether to proceed with the activity.

By its nature, this is a messy activity. Be conscious of protecting clothing and assisting people not to put their hands in their mouths until all paint traces have been removed.

People at the **sensory** level may also enjoy painting to music. The sound of the music, the bright colours and sweeping movements of the hand will stimulate. Again, you may wish to offer hand-over-hand assistance to enable the person to participate in the activity.

DOOR NAMEPLATES

Personalised bedroom doors can help individuals to identify their own room. This can be achieved through colour, door furniture and a nameplate placed in a picture frame at eye level on the door. If the person is involved in the creation of the nameplate it is likely to be easier to identify. This is a very simple and straightforward activity which someone can do on his or her own or as part of a small group.

People who are at the **planned** or **exploratory** activity level can be helped as described below. Those with less ability will need more help and support from an activity worker, key worker, relative or care worker.

You will need to supply a thin card in a range of colours, a variety of paints, pencils, felt tips, and marker pens, scissor and PVA glue.

When inviting people to participate in this activity with you, it may be useful for you to have a completed door nameplate to show them to enable them to understand what you are asking them to do.

Each participant will be asked to pick a background card according to their colour preference. Invite them to write their name on it or perhaps a name they are usually known by or which they prefer to be called. Encourage this to be done in a size large enough to be read from a distance. You could draw a set of parallel lines on the card to facilitate this. Enable the person to decide what coloured medium they would like to use; a mixture of paint and pen is entirely acceptable. You may need to guide the person to write his or her name. Make sure that the paint or pen is completely dry before giving the nameplate to the person. Better still, if you are in a residential establishment, take the person and the nameplate to the person's room to enable him or her to fully complete the activity. (This may be particularly important for people at the **planned** activity level who may be very concerned with the outcome of the activity and would value the opportunity to see it through from beginning to end.)

Added extras...

- Encourage the participants to add pictures by drawing or painting.

- Perhaps add a photograph of the person.

- Have some magazines available and facilitate the person to choose favourite pictures to stick on the nameplate.

- You can use stickers readily available from craft shops to add to the nameplates.

- Consider using glitter and metallic pens for that extra bit of 'bling'.

The person may not wish to put his or her name on the door. Consider options such as 'do not disturb', 'quiet please', 'please knock before entering' or any message the person would like to write.

People at the **exploratory** level will enjoy the process of the activity but may not recollect that the nameplate is for their door. People at the **planned** level will look forward to the outcome as long as they are happy with their completed nameplate.

In either case, if the person does not wish to use the nameplate, do not force the person.

COLLAGE ASSORTMENT PACK AND PVA GLUE

The items in the collage assortment box should be a cacophony of colour, texture and light. You can buy ready-made packs from sources such as the ones at the end of this book, or you can build your own collection. No one could fail to be thrilled and enticed by the glamour of the sequins, the sparkle of the pipe cleaners and ribbons, the fantasy of the feathers.

One gazes into the box with an almost childlike excitement and yearning to feel the items inside. Boxes like this engage the sense of wonder and playfulness in all humans – no matter what the age. This impact alone is reason enough to share the box with the people you care for. We are never too old to imagine or to create. People with cognitive impairments are no less able to call on these skills and concepts, and with careful facilitation can enter a new world of excitement and fantasy.

Unfortunately, collage work has long been associated with either school days or older people sitting around a table with a few odd bits of material and magazines, wishing they were somewhere else! The box in this Activity Pack gives you the opportunity to provide a very different experience of collage work. The skills and opportunities this activity provides for people with cognitive impairments are not only around creativity, but also sharing, communication and teamwork.

For people at the **planned** and **exploratory** activity levels, working on a collage which they have designed and contributed to can be an extremely pleasurable and stimulating experience. Items in this pack will also be of interest to people at a **sensory** or a **reflex** activity level.

By understanding the skills, abilities and preferences of the people you care for, you will be able to identify who would most enjoy participating in this activity. It is important not to mix people from different activity levels. Those at the **planned** level will be very determined about the finished product; what it should look like, where different materials should go, etc. People at the **exploratory** level are likely to be less concerned with the outcome, enjoying the process more. This could lead to some tension within the group particularly if problems arise, which may be difficult for the participants to manage.

As facilitator, you need to monitor the response of each individual group member to ensure that they are enjoying the activity and that they receive recognition for their skills and contribution to the activity. You will need to support participants through any differences of opinion regarding completion of the activity, ensuring that everyone has an opportunity to participate, though some clear leaders may emerge in the group.

If one of the participants has particular expertise in this type of activity, involve them as co-facilitator to maximise opportunities to build their self-esteem.

The running of the group

Make sure that you have an allocated space or room in which to hold the activity. This needs to be interruption free, well lit and ventilated. It is important to consider the skills and expertise of the individuals involved in the activity when deciding how many people to invite into the group. You can do this with just one person, of course, but no more than six people would be optimum.

When inviting participants into the group, it may be useful to have a completed collage or picture to show them or take the box of collage materials to entice them!

The room must be fully prepared for the group's arrival. You will need:

- table and chairs

- a protective cover for the table (e.g. large piece of plastic sheeting)

- large pieces of card that can be taped together once the group has decided how big the collage will be (you could use some sheets of paper from the Creative Activities box)

- the collage box, which contains folds of metallic material, feathers, glitter pipe cleaners, sequin mesh and sequin rows, ribbons, gold and silver braid, holographic and metallic card and paper

- PVA glue, which is decanted into small pots or trays (one for each participant) and glue brush for each participant

- scissors – being mindful of any associated risks.

Additional items which you may wish to provide:

- a selection of magazines, postcards and used greetings cards

- textural items such as cotton wool, string, egg boxes, leaves, dried flower heads, thistles, etc.

- anything which would orientate the group to the season.

Welcome the participants into the group and explain what they will be doing. Share some pictures to enable the group members to begin to identify a theme for their collage.

Suggested themes

- Underwater fantasy
- A day at the seaside
- Holidays
- Countryside
- The seasons
- Theatre night
- Fashion
- Food, glorious food!
- Industry
- The family
- Religious festivals
- High days and holidays
- Favourite things
- Weather

- Light and dark

- Historical events (according to time of year in which anniversary is celebrated)

- Science fiction fantasy.

Once the group have chosen a theme, decide how big the collage will be and adapt your paper or card accordingly. You may wish to complete a rough sketch on the paper, with guidance from the group, as to the positioning of elements of the collage, e.g. sea and sky, land, buildings, trees, etc.

Enable the group to explore all the different materials available. Some decisions will begin to be made about which material would suit which element of the collage. Put the material/s on the rough design according to where it will positioned in the final collage.

You may like to allocate specific activities to the individual group members, with their agreement. This will be particularly helpful to people at the **planned** activity level who will appreciate clearly identified activities which they can complete before moving on to the next activity. People at the **exploratory** level will enjoy one-step activities but may require additional support and guidance to maintain focus and momentum.

Suggested tasks

- Collecting suitable materials (e.g. of same colour/texture)

- Cutting chosen material into shapes

- Gluing material onto collage

- Working on specific element of collage (e.g. sky, sea, figures, etc.)

- Working on specific area of collage (e.g. bottom/top corner, left/right side)

- Overseeing the whole collage, keeping people on track, keeping image of finished collage in mind, referring to picture if being used as guide.

Play some gentle music, related to the theme if possible, in the background as people work. Encourage interaction and sharing, decision making, reminiscence and laughter. Constantly monitor the response of the individuals. Have a tea or coffee break at an appropriate moment and allow the participants to reflect on the work so far.

You will need to decide whether the collage will need to be finished in one session. Can you arrange another session with the participants? Can you leave it out safely for participants to work on at their leisure? Do you have somewhere you can store the 'work in progress' and all the materials? Make sure that you have safely disposed of any glue which has not been used.

Always thank the participants for joining in with the activity and for their contribution. Specifically highlight one thing for each individual that has impressed you and tell them so, as part of the group reflection. Ask the group participants what they have enjoyed.

Ultimately decide with the participants where the collage will be hung. An unveiling ceremony might be fun, if the 'collage makers' are in agreement.

More ideas...

You could facilitate individuals to complete their own collage. Enable them to choose the size of paper to work on; A4 may be suitable. They can choose their materials and theme and work on this independently or among a group of others who are all working on their own collages.

The collages could remain individual or the participants may be agreeable for them to be stuck together, particularly if they have all been working on the same theme.

People at the **sensory** activity level might enjoy the collage pack in a different way. They may be able to contribute to the completion of collage, given verbal and physical guidance on a one-to-one basis throughout. They may, more simply, enjoy exploring the contents of the box, feeling the different textures and seeing the different colours and sparkle. This relates well to the sort of sensory work that really stimulates people at this activity level.

You could also select specific items from the box that have an interesting texture, a strong colour or some sparkle and share them, one at a time, with people at a **reflex** level. Some lurex material placed in the palm of the hand may elicit a grasp response and a feather in a bright colour stroked on the back of the hand may be of interest to the person.

It is essential that the collage facilitators are enthusiastic about this activity and have some skill themselves. This will help to generate ideas and identify the process, contributing significantly to the design. If you have access to the Internet there are some fascinating websites specifically on collage and ideas. Put 'collage ideas' into your search engine.

MODELLING DOUGH AND MODELLING SET

Creativity and art is all about stimulating the senses and freeing the mind. Mankind has used sculpture as an artistic medium for thousands of years, again in veneration of deities, recording of historical events and expression of the self.

As children we often enjoyed the tactile sensation of clay and plasticine and the myriad forms we could make from it. As we grew older, we used clay and other pliable materials to make three-dimensional figures or things we could use: mugs, boxes, badges, jewellery. A gift which someone had made was always a delight to receive. For some this enjoyment has become a much-loved hobby or a business.

Whether for play or for profit, using and modelling clay or dough enables us to use and develop a variety of skills that are transferable. For example, modelling dough can be replaced with pastry dough.

The benefits of using modelling dough with people with cognitive impairments

- Emphasis is on use of the senses, particularly touch and vision.

- Straightforward series of single steps to achieve outcome.

- Quick results can engage concentration and attention skills.

- Familiar patterns of movement may be elicited.

- Memories evoked can lead to reminiscence.

- Opportunity to learn or re-establish a skill.

- Provides opportunity for communication and social interaction – verbal and nonverbal.

- Exercises joints and muscles of hands.

- Facilitates use of imagination and play.

- Errors can be turned into successes quickly and easily.

- Opportunity to experience a sense of achievement.

- Opportunity to transfer skills learnt in other types of activity (e.g. baking).

Be careful to present this activity appropriately so that people do not feel that you are treating them childishly.

People at the **planned** activity level may enjoy modelling the dough, being conscious of complex uses for it with definite end results in mind: figurines, models of animals, etc. They may wish to use the different coloured doughs on a single piece (e.g. modelling a bowl of fruit or bunch of flowers). This may lead them onto modelling with air-hardening dough or salt dough to achieve a more lasting result.

The modelling dough can be used for people at the **exploratory** and **sensory** activity levels. What is most engaging about this activity is the effect upon the senses, which will be really motivating for the participants. The colours are bright, the dough smells wonderful and the feel of it as it is moulded in the hands is relaxing and soothing.

One of the aims of this activity is to enable people to use choice: to pick the colour dough they want to work with, to mould an object of their choice or just to handle the dough. People may not have an idea what they want to mould until they actually start handling the dough. For people at these activity levels it is not necessary to pursue an 'end result', though they might surprise themselves with a skill they did not know they had!

Enable participants to handle the dough and use the modelling set too. The modelling set typically consists of rolling pins, spatulas and a variety of dough cutters. You can buy these as sets or obtain items individually.

Facilitate the participants to use some of these items to explore the dough even more. People at the **sensory** level may need hand-over-hand assistance to do this. Constantly monitor the response of the participants, to ensure that they are enjoying the activity and sensation of the dough in their hands. Once finished with, the dough can be remoulded and shaped back into tubes to be placed in the plastic bags for use next time. Try to ensure mixed colours of dough are taken apart before remoulding.

Be conscious of whether the person would like to keep the object they have made.

PRECAUTIONS

Please be advised that the colour on the dough does come off on the hands. This is easily washed off with soap and water. You will need to consider protecting clothes in case someone rubs their hands over them, but again the colour will wash out.

Be aware that people may take the dough to their mouths and may try to eat it. Please support participants to prevent this from happening as part of your risk assessment of the person and activity.

The dough is nontoxic, but if some is eaten, you may wish to seek medical advice.

SUMMARY

Art activities provide a wonderful way to enable people at all activity levels to express themselves; it should also be good fun too.

You will always be guided by the needs, preferences and response of the individuals you are working with. Facilitators are required to be knowledgeable and enthusiastic too, to really maximise opportunities for engagement and a sense of purpose.

Be mindful always of how you present the activity in order that it meets the activity level of the person *now*, not what it may have been some years ago. Also be aware of how you assess and manage the risks associated with using paint and coloured pens.

Lastly, always be encouraging, reassuring and supportive. A facilitator's role is not to criticise, not to 'correct', not to pass judgement. It is to facilitate, enable and empower.

Chapter 14

Sensory Activities Pack

SUGGESTED CONTENTS

- Relaxation Music CD
- Rainmaker
- Doll
- Footspa
- Coloured light sphere lamp
- Vibrating pillow
- Bumpie ball
- Lavender moisturising body lotion

INTRODUCTION

This pack will be appropriate for those at all levels of ability using the Pool Activity Level (PAL) Instrument.

Most of the objects in this pack are intended to be used in individual activity sessions with the carer. It is possible that some may also be used in a small group, but the carer will need to observe each participant and judge if all are gaining something from the activity. The length of time each activity lasts will, again, be determined by the individual's response to the object, and will rely on the carer's observational skills to determine when the activity should cease. People with moderate to severe cognitive impairments may have a very short attention span and the activity may only be appropriate for a few minutes. In these cases it is best to use a 'little and often' approach.

UNDERSTANDING THE ABILITY OF THE PERSON

Understanding what the person can and cannot do is vital to the success of the activity. If an activity is too difficult, a person may become anxious or frustrated. If the activity is too easy, the person may feel unmotivated to take part.

A person who has moderate to severe impairments is likely to be responding to his or her world mainly through the senses, even in a purely reflex response to specific stimuli. When we know this, we can help the person to engage with the world by presenting sensations to the person. Therefore some of the activities in this pack are particularly beneficial for people at a **sensory** or a **reflex** level.

SENSORY ACTIVITY LEVEL

At a **sensory** activity level the person may not have many thoughts or ideas about carrying out an activity; he or she is mainly concerned with the sensation and with moving his or her body in response to those sensations. People at this level can be guided to carry out single-step activities such as sweeping or winding wool. More complex activities can only be carried out when directed one step at a time. Therefore care givers need to ensure that the person at this activity level has the opportunity to experience a wide variety of sensations, and to carry out one-step activities. Directions to maximise this opportunity need to be kept very simple and to be reinforced by demonstrating the action required.

REFLEX ACTIVITY LEVEL

A person at a **reflex** activity level may not be aware of the surrounding environment or even of his or her own body. He or she is living in a subliminal or subconscious state, where movement is a reflex response to a stimulus. Therefore people wishing to enter into this person's consciousness need to use direct sensory stimulation. By using direct stimulation the person's self-awareness can be raised. A person at this level may have difficulty in organising more than one sensation that is being experienced at the same time. Excessive or multiple stimuli can cause distress; therefore crowds, loud noises, and background clamour should be avoided. Activities at this level should focus on introducing a single sensation to the person. A care giver interacting with a person at a **reflex** level needs to use all his or her communication skills to enter into the world of a person at this level. Language skills tend to play only a minor role at this level and should be kept to single words, although the use of facial expression and of a warm and reassuring tone and volume can be vital in establishing a communication channel.

RELAXATION MUSIC CD

Music is a very personal choice but it touches most of us with its ability to enhance mood and well-being. The rhythm and beat of music can have a direct effect on the physical functions of the body; a slow rhythm influences the heart to beat more slowly and leads to a sense of calm and relaxation. There are many CDs of this type available from most music shops.

There are several ways that this CD might be used. It may form the end of a more invigorating activity, such as a group game or a movement to music session that encourages mobility. Some ideas for this are presented below. Alternatively, the CD may be used simply as a relaxation activity in a group or individually for people who need help to relax.

Relaxation technique

Make sure that everyone is sitting comfortably; that their head and arms are supported and that their feet are firmly on the floor.

For people who are able to imitate movement and to follow instructions (**sensory**, **exploratory** and **planned** levels) demonstrate the following actions and encourage them to copy you. Reinforce people's involvement with smiles and nods.

- Tighten the muscles in your toes. Hold for a count of ten. Relax and enjoy the sensation of release from tension.

- Flex the muscles in your feet. Hold for a count of ten. Relax.

- Move slowly up through your body – legs, abdomen, back, neck, face – contracting and relaxing muscles as you go.

- Now close your eyes and listen to the music while you breathe deeply and slowly.

- Finally stop the music, ask everyone to open their eyes and encourage them to gently stretch and to look around them.

Thank everyone for joining in and ask if they would like to do the activity again at another time.

You will need to make more direct contact with people who are unable to imitate movement and to follow instructions (**reflex** level). This is likely to be a one-to-one activity. Sit next to and slightly to one side of the person and gently and firmly hold the person's hands. Make eye contact and smile and nod, say 'listen' and 'lovely' and breathe deeply. Stroke the back of the person's hand, using firm and gentle movements that are in time with the beat of the music.

Movement to music

Select music with a strong, fairly fast beat. Make sure people who are at risk of falling are seated. Hand out two brightly coloured scarves to each person and keep two to yourself. Begin to wave them in time to the music and encourage others to join in. Play two fast tunes.

Now play the Relaxation Music CD and encourage everyone to listen to it and to relax.

Variations

1.   Use a large cloth or parachute to get everyone to hold. This forms a connection with each other, and may be useful for people who are more impaired (**reflex** level) and need more help to make movements.

2.   For people who can imitate actions of another person (**sensory**, **exploratory** or **planned** levels) lead everyone to move different parts of the body, starting with the shoulders:

   - shoulders: shrugging and relaxing

   - arms: straight out in front and moving to the side and back

   - straight out in front and raising up and down

   - out to each side and turning small circles

   - hands: miming playing the piano

   - turning the wrists and hands over and back

   - waist: leaning forwards while holding onto the chair arms

   - turning to the left and then to the right, holding onto the chair arms

   - legs: stamping feet up and down

   - knees: straightening and bending

   - ankles: pointing feet to the ceiling and down to the floor

   - drawing circles with the toes.

RAINMAKER

The traditional rainsticks originated in northern Chile where they are used in ceremonies to bring rain. Made from the skeleton of the capado cactus when it dies, it is dried, hollowed out, and filled with small seeds or pebbles. Small nails are driven through the hull of the cactus in a spiral formation, and when the rainstick is inverted the filling striking the nails creates the sound of water falling.

Commercially available rainmakers come in a variety of sizes, materials and colours, from plastic ones filled with brightly coloured beads to wooden ones, all designed to enables users to enjoy watching, hearing and feeling the 'rain' fall. By holding it straight up and down or angled, you can create anything from a hurricane to a gentle spring shower. Plastic rainmakers have special prisms in the walls of the instrument to create a rainbow of colours as the beads cascade through the tube. Those with a rubber ring exterior help to give an easy grip when used.

The rainmaker is intended for use by people with severe cognitive impairments (**reflex** level) who will be engaging with their world through the senses of touch, hearing and sight. It can help the person to focus on an object and to sustain attention for a few moments.

Show the person the rainmaker and invert it to show the person how it works. Use smiles and nods and say 'listen' and 'look' to show the person what is happening.

Offer the rainmaker to the person. Help the person to hold and move the rainmaker (you may need to hold your hand over theirs).

This may be an activity of only a few moments. Carefully observe the response of the person by looking at his or her body language, particularly facial expression and posture. Remove the rainmaker if the person responds negatively to it or begins to lose interest.

Leave the rainmaker with the person if he or she engages positively with it. If the person takes the rainmaker to his or her mouth to explore it, encourage this to happen. Clean the rainmaker after with a mild antibacterial solution.

Finish by thanking the person for taking part (even if the person does not seem to know what you are saying, the tone of your voice will be important).

DOLLS

Dolls have long been recognised as an integral part of human development and play throughout the centuries and across cultures. Children have longed for the 'doll of the year' at Christmas time and adult collectors have longed for the exquisite 'limited edition doll'.

When working with people with cognitive impairment the use of dolls provides us with the opportunity to explore the many facets of a human being in terms of emotional expression, communication, attachment, development and playfulness.

Therapeutic dolls are commercially available. You may wish to dress the doll or have a variety of clothing available for it.

For people who have moderate to severe cognitive impairments (**sensory** and **reflex** level), the doll may be used to assist in the enhancement of well-being as well as to provide an opportunity for the person to engage in meaningful interaction, expression of emotion and demonstration of the role 'mother' or 'father'.

It is not always necessary or appropriate to directly give a person the doll in the first instance. Place the doll within the visual field of the person and use verbal, nonverbal and sensory cues to direct the person toward the doll. The cue may be the texture of the doll's garment or skin, the colour of the garment, or smell (rub a little talcum powder onto the doll).

Carefully monitor the person's response, particularly facial expression. The person may smile at the doll or reach out for it. If this happens place the doll on the person's lap or in the cradle of the person's elbow.

Continue to monitor the response of the person closely. The person may rock the doll, speak to it or sing. If the person is singing, join in gently and quietly. Encourage the person to stroke the doll. He or she may wish to play with the doll's garments, or remove them. Again, join in with positive verbal and nonverbal responses, constantly monitoring the response of the person.

Leave the doll with the person if he or she engages positively with it. If the person begins to lose interest in the doll or it is ignored, remove the doll, thanking the person for joining you in that moment.

As with all activities, it is essential that you have a good biography of the person before you engage in working with the doll. A doll can be a highly emotive symbol of love or pain, of parenthood or the yearning for parenthood, of success or loss.

You will know from the person's biography what response *may* be elicited when working with the doll. However, do not make assumptions about gender and do not assume that someone who enjoyed dolls many years ago will do so now. Do not exclude an individual from a potentially positive experience in the assumption that the person did not like dolls in the past.

Be mindful of your own attitudes and feelings about dolls and the therapeutic use of dolls. This is an opportunity to be truly person centred and to possibly enter a humbling, enriched world.

THE FOOTSPA

Footspas are available from a variety of sources including chemists and supermarkets. They will come with comprehensive instructions, which *you must follow at all times*.

The footspa can be used with people at both **sensory** and **reflex** level.

It is important to follow the preparation guidelines as it can take a short while to set up the footspa – you do not want to lose an opportunity to engage a person in this activity if his or her attention is lost early on.

As with all the activities it is important that you know the person well. You need to consider how the person responds to touch, whether he or she likes water, how he or she responds to noise and vibration, whether he or she likes the feet being touched.

You might want to consider introducing the use of the footspa as part of an individual's self-care routine. It is important that you introduce this activity slowly and with sensitivity.

Ensure that the person is seated in an upright chair to maintain good posture and optimum positioning to enable the person to engage fully. The person may like to have someone sitting alongside them for reassurance and affirmation.

Remove the person's shoes and socks/stockings/tights. Reinforce this by explaining to the person what you are doing. (The person may not understand your words but will appreciate your reassuring, calm tone.)

Gently rub or stroke the person's feet for a few moments to enable them to begin to identify with the sensory stimulus and assist with orientation to that part of the body.

Introduce the footspa slowly. Perhaps you could drip a little water over the person's feet to enable him or her to experience a changed sensation. Carefully monitor the person's response. If the person shows negative response signs, grimaces or cries out, then withdraw the foot, change posture, end the activity immediately and offer reassurance. If the person remains calm, shows positive signs, smiles, laughs, and offers attention: continue.

Gently place the person's feet – one at a time – into the footspa. Again, continually monitor the person's response. Gently massage the feet in the water allowing the water to gently splash. Use verbal and nonverbal communication throughout: eye contact, smiling, 'ooh' and 'aah', 'how nice'.

Continue to monitor the response and, if the person appears to be enjoying the sensation, consider changing the setting of the footspa:

- whirl and heat

- massage only

- whirl, heat and massage.

Remember that too much sensory stimulus can cause distress, so carefully monitor the response at each stage.

You may wish to use the Relaxation Music CD in this pack as gentle background music while the person enjoys the activity.

Check the temperature of the water at all times; do not allow it to become too hot or cold.

Monitoring the response of the person, agree when the activity is complete. Carefully lift the feet – one at a time – out of the footspa and remove it to a safe distance. Gently towel dry the person's feet, again monitoring his or her response and reinforcing your actions with verbal and nonverbal communication.

Apply talcum powder or moisturiser if required. Replace socks/tights/stockings and shoes.

Sit quietly with the person for a few moments, talk about the activity and thank the person for joining in.

COLOURED LIGHT SPHERE

A coloured light sphere can be used with people at both **sensory** and **reflex** levels.

The use of slow-moving light can help to rehabilitate some of the visual skills of a person with cognitive impairment. When used therapeutically, with another person's facilitation, the lamp can help the person to focus attention on, and to track movement of, the multicoloured light rays.

Use of the coloured light sphere can also help to reduce stress-related behaviour. You may wish to use the Relaxation Music CD in this pack as gentle background music while the person enjoys the activity.

Introduce the person to the coloured light sphere while it is switched off. Describe what it will do – 'This ball will give off lots of different coloured lights' – and ask if the person would like to see it: 'Would you like to see?'. Explain that you are going to switch it on and when the rays begin to move use your verbal and nonverbal communication skills to facilitate the person to see them: 'Look', 'Watch', 'See the red one'. Use the person's name also to stimulate his or her attention to your communication and use pointing to help direct his or her gaze.

Carefully monitor the person's response to the moving light rays. If the person shows negative response signs – which may include withdrawal, rocking, tense posture, or crying out – end the activity immediately and offer reassurance.

If the person remains calm, shows positive signs, smiles, laughs, and offers attention: continue. You may find it helpful, once the person's attention has been captured, to remain silent and enable the person to enjoy the experience.

Monitoring the response of the person, agree when the activity is complete. Switch off the coloured light sphere and sit quietly with the person for a few moments, talk about the activity and thank the person for joining in.

VIBRATING PILLOW

Vibrating pillows are available from some of the sources listed at the start of this chapter. They will come with comprehensive instructions, which *you must follow at all times*.

The vibrating pillow can be used with people at both **sensory** and **reflex** levels. Users at a **sensory** level will be able to activate the vibrations and turn them off themselves. This can give a sense of control over one's own environment and a sense of achievement in making something happen. The vibrating pillow is also useful for people functioning at a **reflex** level who may have difficulty initiating any movement of their own and rely on direct stimulation of the senses in order to make a movement in response.

The sensation of vibration can offer powerful stimulation as well as a means of keeping the person's attention and calming troubled behaviour. The vibrating pillow is made from a tactile fabric, which the person can be encouraged to stroke and smooth as an introduction to this activity.

Explain to the person that this pillow can vibrate and show them what happens when you apply pressure to start the vibrations and release pressure for the vibrations to stop. Use your own body language, smiling and nodding, to give the message that this is acceptable and enjoyable and use spoken language: 'ooh', 'aah', 'lovely'.

Encourage people at a **sensory** level to apply pressure and to release it themselves and acknowledge when they have achieved it: 'Well done, it's working', 'Good for you, it's switched off'. Encourage people to experiment with experiencing the vibrations through the hands, back, stomach, feet.

Assist the person at a **reflex** level to apply pressure, or place it in a position where pressure is naturally applied: behind the small of the back or under the feet.

Carefully monitor the person's response to the vibrations. If the person shows negative response signs – which may include withdrawal, rocking, tense posture, or crying out – end the activity immediately and offer reassurance.

If the person remains calm, shows positive signs, smiles, laughs, and offers attention: continue. You may find it helpful, once the person's attention has been captured, to remain silent and enable the person to enjoy the experience.

Monitoring the response of the person, agree when the activity is complete. Remove the vibrating pillow and sit quietly with the person for a few moments, talk about the activity and thank the person for joining in.

The person must not be left unaccompanied with this vibrating pillow, as prolonged sensory stimulation may be uncomfortable and distressing.

BUMPIE BALL

The 'interestingly' named Bumpie Ball can be used with people at both **sensory** and **reflex** activity levels. The texture, colour, shape of the ball can be extremely attractive and a little intriguing.

People at the **sensory** activity level will be able to grasp the ball and can be encouraged to explore its facets. People at a **reflex** level can be stimulated by the ball when used as a massager.

Offer the ball to the person who is at the **sensory** activity level. You may present it as an 'interesting object' which you would like to share and explore with the person.

Allow the person to take the ball and wait a few moments to see how he or she responds. If the person's attention is drawn to the ball, the person looks at it or perhaps moves it around on his or her hand, reinforce this response with positive comments, for example: 'it feels nice', 'it's soft', 'what a lovely colour'.

Encourage the person to sense the ball through sight and touch. Allow the person to explore the ball with both hands. The person may pick at the bumps on the ball or stroke it. Accompany this with calm, reassuring comments, constantly monitoring the person's response.

The person may take the ball to their mouth. (You can wash the ball after it has been used.)

The person may throw the ball toward you or pass it back to you. Facilitate this opportunity for turn taking and promoting a sense of agency by returning the ball to the person, either a gentle throw or placing in the person's hands or lap. Maintain eye contact with the person, smile and mirror the person's positive responses.

It may be possible to engage with more than one person, by passing or throwing the ball to others in combination with saying their name. It is *vital* that you ensure that you have gained the attention of the person before throwing or even passing the ball to him or her. The person must be prepared to receive the ball, otherwise they will be startled and distressed.

Constantly monitor the response of the person. The person may throw the ball away, or he or she may be unresponsive or uninterested in the ball, allowing it to sit in his or her lap without touching it. In this instance remove the ball and consider offering a different type of stimulus according to the person's preference.

If the person does show interest in the ball and appears stimulated by it, you may consider including the ball in a 'Feely Bag' containing other objects such as a silk scarf, fur, cotton wool, a necklace of beads, which you can take out in turn for the person to touch and explore. The person might enjoy watching you blow the ball up, engaging with their sense of hearing – and fun!

For a person who is at the **reflex** activity level, the Bumpie Ball can be used as a massager.

Ensure that you have gained the attention of the person; seek eye contact or movement toward you in recognition of your voice or touch to their hand or shoulder. The person should be seated in an upright chair and in a good position.

Place the ball in the person's lap and lift one of his or her hands on top of it. Constantly monitor the response of the person. If the person cries out or withdraws his or her hand, remove the ball immediately and give reassurance.

By studying the person's positive nonverbal responses, continue with the activity by placing your hand over his or her hand and gently moving the ball in rhythmic patterns.

If the person is willing and responds positively, take the ball from under the person's hand and gently roll it up his or her arm. Continuously monitor the response of the person as you roll the ball up the arm and across the back of the shoulders and gently down the other arm. It is hoped that the sensation of pressure will be stimulating for the person or an enjoyable, relaxing experience. (It will be helpful to have a colleague with you so that they can monitor the person's response as you roll the ball across his or her shoulders.)

You may wish to use the Relaxation Music CD included in this pack to reinforce the gentle, relaxing atmosphere.

Again, your knowledge of the person, and constant monitoring of his or her response, will guide you as to whether to place the ball under the person's feet. Sit at the person's feet, ensuring that you have gained his or her attention. Gently remove the shoe from one of his or her feet and massage the foot to enable the person to recognise the stimulation to that part of the body. Lift the foot and place it on top of the ball. Holding gently to the foot and lower limb, allow the limb to move rhythmically as the ball sways and moves beneath. Repeat with the other foot, constantly monitoring the person's response.

If the person cries out, withdraws the limb or expresses ill-being, remove the ball immediately, allowing the foot to rest gently back into position and offer reassurance.

Monitoring the response of the person, agree when the activity has ended. Replace the person's shoes and perhaps sit quietly with him or her or listen to the Relaxation Music CD.

Thank the person for joining in the activity with you and ensure that the person is aware that the activity is ended.

LAVENDER MOISTURISING BODY LOTION

We interact with the environment and people around us through stimulation of our senses. When people are asked 'Which of the senses would you least like to lose?' they often have difficulty in deciding. It is difficult to imagine such a loss and the impact this would have on our life and abilities.

In working with people with cognitive impairments we have the opportunity of engaging and communicating in a variety of ways, not least through the sense of smell.

It must be remembered that not everyone has the same experience of smell, that this sense may be damaged through neurological impairment or the normal ageing process. Some people may never have had a sense of smell; for some this may have been heightened.

In terms of orientation, smell is invaluable. For many, the smell of pine, cinnamon and spiced fruit will make them think of Christmas. Who can smell freshly cut grass or a sea breeze without thinking of summer?

Memory and the sense of smell are both associated with the function of the temporal lobe in the brain. It is not surprising that there is such a close relationship.

Lavender has long been considered one of the most recognisable of smells. It has associations with clean, crisp linen, lavender bags, perfume and even sweets. Many people have grown lavender in their garden and immediately recognise its aroma. Latterly, the benefits of lavender as an essential oil have been recognised in terms of relaxation and healing. While essential oils can be contra-indicated for some people and should only be used by qualified aromatherapists, it is possible to gain some benefits from moisturisers and lotions that contain these oils. Lavender moisturising body lotion recommended for this pack can be used with people at both **sensory** and **reflex** activity levels.

As with all activities, it is essential to know the person's history, their likes and dislikes and in this instance whether they have a sense of smell! (In this case you would adapt the activity accordingly.)

For a person at the **sensory** level the body lotion can be used in a variety of ways, depending upon their response.

Show the person the body lotion bottle, informing them that there is lavender-scented lotion in it. This may elicit an immediate response. The person may take the bottle from you. If the person would like to remove the lid, encourage the person to do so or offer the necessary support to assist him or her.

Encourage the person to smell the lotion in the bottle. Make sure that they do not breathe in too deeply or frequently as this may cause them to feel dizzy/hyperventilate. You smell it too.

Encourage communication – 'what a lovely smell', 'what does that remind you of?', 'mmm, how lovely', 'do you like it?'. Use nonverbal communication too: smiling, closing eyes and exaggerating inhalation, maintain eye contact. The person may be able to spontaneously reminisce; encourage this with open questions and reflection.

Of course the person may not be able to smell it, so do not labour the above. They also may not like the smell or it may hold negative associations – be prepared for this.

Ask if the person would like to have some lotion placed on his or her hand. If so, ensure that the person's clothing is protected by rolling up sleeves and placing a towel over the lap. The person may pour lotion into his or her hands spontaneously and begin to massage it. Again, reinforce this with positive communication, talking about how it feels, reinforcing reminiscence, recognising that the smell may become more pungent.

If the person does not put lotion onto his or her hands, ask if you can do this for the person. Constantly monitor the person's response. Be aware of the temperature of the lotion as it may be quite cold when coming directly from the bottle.

In both cases, constantly monitor the person's response. Ask if the person would like you to give him or her a hand massage. If they agree, the following massage guide may be useful.

1. Ensure that you have adequate moisturising lotion on your hands. Carefully rub your hands together to warm the lotion.

2. Take the person's hand in yours and, holding it palm down, use your thumbs to gently massage the back of the hand.

3. Turn the hand over and gently massage the palm with your thumbs.

4. Palm to palm, use circular movements over the person's hand and fingers.

5. Massage each digit in turn, starting with the thumb and continuing, finishing with the little finger.

6. Use stroking movements over the palm and back of the hand, extending up over the wrist to midway between wrist and elbow.

7. Circle the hand and wrist with your hands using rhythmical, gentle upward and downward, flowing movements as your hands overlap.

8. Use downward stroking movements over the back and palm of the person's hand.

9. The massage is complete.

10. Use a towel to remove any excess lotion.

Thank the person for participating in the activity with you and ask the person how he or she feels. Sit quietly with the person before formally ending the activity.

You could use the body lotion as a resource for a small group of people, all at the **sensory** level, by developing an 'olfactory stimulation kit' or 'smelly box'.

Transfer items such as the body lotion, coffee essence, washing powder, mint mouthwash, brandy, herbs, vinegar, into lidded containers.

Present the activity as a 'smell quiz', allowing participants to smell each item in turn, to see if they can identify it and reminisce.

For people at the **reflex** level, you can use the body lotion in the same way as for the hand massage activity. Make sure that you continuously monitor the response of the individual and adjust the activity accordingly. You may also wish to use the body lotion in conjunction with the footspa included in this pack.

Play the Relaxation Music CD to accompany the massage if appropriate, but be careful not to offer too much sensory stimulation as this can be distressing for the individual.

Ensure that participants do not attempt to ingest the contents of the containers and that they do not hyperventilate.

Suppliers

Baker Ross Ltd

2–3 Forest Works

Forest Road

Walthamstow

London E17 6JG

www.bakerross.co.uk

The Consortium

Hammond Way

Trowbridge

Wiltshire BA14 8RR

www.theconsortium.co.uk

Hobbycraft (stores located in England and Wales)

Head Office

7 Enterprise Way

Aviation Park

Bournemouth International Airport

Christchurch

Dorset BH23 6HG

www.hobbycraft.co.uk

Nottingham Rehab Supplies

Nottingham Logistics Centre

Victoria Business Park

Pintail Close

Netherfield

Nottingham NG4 2PE

www.nrs-uk.co.uk

ROMPA

Goyt Side Road

Chesterfield

Derbyshire S40 2PH

www.rompa.com

TFH Special Needs Toys

5–7 Severnside Business Park

Severn Road

Stourport-on-Severn

Worcestershire DY13 9HT

www.tfhuk.com

Winslow

Goyt Side Road

Chesterfield

Derbyshire S40 2PH

www.winslow-cat.com